Long Hard Road

Ruth Macklin

Chapter One

Free! If only I were free! Free to spread my wings wide and be able to fly. Fly on the wind and soar above the land, across the oceans through out the world. To wonder over hill and dale. See all the wonders of the world then return home to my new home, home to my own castle, Castle of Angels. The turrets would have statues of angels across the front of the castle. There would be a mosaic of an angel either side of the front door. The door would have stained glass inlaid into the wood. A front porch with Roman columns to hold up the roof to keep the sun, and the rain, away from the front door.

Because of the Australian hot sun the castle would have to be built with a wide veranda as most of the old Queensland style homes did but glassed in to protect anyone resting on the veranda from the different elements of the weather.

In the entry way would be a round cement pond covered with aquamarine tile on both the inside and around the out side. In the middle of the pond would be a fountain with an angel on the top with water spraying from the head to fall back into the water at the gold fish pond. Gold fish would glide through the water beneath the water lily leaves floating on the surface of the water. Lights of different shades, changing to different colours as they flashed on the Angel spraying out the water.

My castle would have to be about three stories high to accommodate all the rooms I wished to have to be able to spread out all my belongings, so I would be able to find

them, not have to search the house to find the items which I needed. At the moment I

have started building my castle in my mind until the day when I can afford to build it for

real. To let the world know that I have arrived. I had rose to the top of the world by

crawling my way from a nothing to a very powerful woman. A woman where everyone

beat a path to my door for guidance, help, because I would be rich in all areas of my life. I

wouldn't need to worry where to find my next feed. Won't have to worry that I am unable

to do all the work I would like to be able to do. I will be able to do what I would like to

do for a change. Just like the birds I would be able to travel to where the weather is more

suitable, not too hot, or too cold. If all my friends in the outer universe keep looking out

for my welfare I WILL make my dreams of owning my own castle come true.

As I have a slowly growing family, I would have to have a lot of rooms, or suites, or

family sections, where there were a number of rooms, a bath room with a bath, shower,

wash basin, and cupboards for the towels and other items needed for use in the bathroom;

a toilet. The floors in the bathroom would be tiled in the colour scheme to suit the room.

Curtains to match and a couple of plants which would be able to survive in side and in a

steamy environment. There would also need to be a small kitchen to provide food and

drink, in each room so the occupant would not have to traverse through the castle in

search of what they wanted. There would have to be a small fridge, table and chairs,

electric jug to boil water for a hot drink, cupboards for china and nibbles. All furniture

Ruth Macklin

except the bed would be built in so there would be no need to move too much when cleaning the rooms. There would be a couple of lazy-boy chairs for someone to sit and read if they wanted some peace, or just to while away the time if they could not sleep.

The bedrooms would have to be on the first floor reached by a wide staircase which went up to a small landing, with a branch to left and right, to take you to different sections of the castle. Then there would have to be other stairs from each level to reach the other floors. There would have to be at least four family areas, ten or more, other rooms with en suites, also with kitchenette and small lounge area.

The next level up would be mine. There would be a bedroom for me with en suite, a walk-in wardrobe, a duchess and bed. A fully equipped small kitchen so I could eat there if I were busy and didn't want to be disturbed. Or disturb anyone if I want to work late at night. A small lounge room where I could sit and relax to while away the stress of daily life; to recoup my strength for the coming new day.

A very large study with desks for working on, computers, printers, scanners, fax and telephone. Some filing cabinets and shelves with glassed in fronts in which to keep all the books I might need for some of my work. A place to set up my music. A CD player and cassette for playing music. Cupboards to store such things as paper, cartridges for the printer, and other office supplies. A large table to set out my work so I could find it. A small water feature where the water sound would have a calming effect on me as I worked..

Ruth Macklin

There would be a room for all my craft materials so I can go in there to work on my craft when I need time for thinking, or relaxing. Where I could crochet, knit, do tatting, or any other craft I may feel like doing to keep the fingers working, to stop the mind from vegetating. A vault would also be on the same floor where I could keep all important document and other items of value from being destroyed by fire, or damaged by an act or nature; or stolen.

Up on the roof which would be cement there would be tables and chairs for people to relax in the sun, or moonlight. A look out to make sure the castle and the surrounding area was safe from any advancing fire front. There would be a fire hose placed in each corner of the roof to protect the castle from fire and keep the surrounding area wet to stop it catching fire. There would be a small room for a desk with a phone so valuable time would not be lost in getting help. Another place to be alone if I needed to think late at night with not a worry about the weather be it hot, cold, or wet. A quiet place where I could communicate with all the powers from above in the universe, to be able to look at the moon and stars which is impossible to do most of the time while living in the city. The lights on the streets and in the houses which blocked out the shine of the stars.

There would be a elevator so it would be easier for the elder generation of visitors, or handicapped, to be able to make it up to the bedrooms in comfort instead of trying to struggle up the stairs. To be also use for getting all the furniture up to the next levels. Make the work easier on the persons doing the hard work so there would be no one

Ruth Macklin

getting hurt.

Also, on my floor, I would like a special room where I would be able to go to meditate to relieve the stress, cleanse the body of unhealthy thoughts, hassles and pain. To recharge my body for the coming day. A place which would be free from the troubles of the outside world, my haven to cast away all danger with spells. To be able to pray to the Angels for help to remove the problems which have been causing trouble for my family. Make everything easier for me to fulfil all the things I wish to accomplish for those around me and make life easier, and healthier, for one and all. A place where I could talk to my Angels who have been constantly with me to show me the way I should travel.

On the ground floor there would be a very large cooking area with cupboards to store all the equipment where it would be easy to reach, and easy to find. A big pantry to store some of the food and a cold room to store boxes of cold foods, that way we would not have to go into town on frequent trips to buy just a few things. There would be stoves which use electricity and gas so if one is not available, there is still some way of cooking food. Fridges for the food which were in daily use. Plenty of bench space for the preparation of the food. Dishwasher and a couple of sinks for the cleaning up of the dishes.

There would be a large dinning room with tables and chairs. Cupboards to store the china and cutlery, glasses, and other dishes which would be need to be used to decorate the tables. In the middle of the room there would hang a chandelier as well as smaller

Ruth Macklin

lights in scones on the walls, that could be brightened, or dimmed, to suit the occasion.

A sun room would be another place where anyone could go to rest, or talk. For anyone else who might like to go there to be among the plants which would be in the room if they didn't want to go out side in the hot, bright sun; or couldn't walk around out side. In one corner would be a small water feature. Most of the water features would be for calming, and cooling the castle to help save on energy use.

At one section of the castle would be a ballroom type room where people could have a wedding breakfast if they so desired, or a conference. It would have a chandelier each end of the room with scones around the walls. A small stage where there could be a band or singers, to entertain the guests. A piano and an organ would be there for those who just wanted music for entertainment, or dancing. Rest rooms and toilets for the people so they would not have to wander through the private section of the castle. It would have to be sound proofed so that the music, or any noise, would not disturb the rest of the people in the castle.

There would be a working office for the running of all the programs which would be held at the castle. Where bookings could be made for the use of the ballroom; visiting the gardens; or just a place to holiday.

A library would be another room I would need to store all the books I have acquired over the years which most of them are at the moment stored in boxes, and cupboards. I am quickly running out of room to hide them out of the way. There would have to be two

Ruth Macklin

walls at least with glassed in front doors to protect the books from damage, and dust.

Then a photo room would be good to display all the family photos, and paintings, which can't be done at the moment. Some photos I can't hang because the unseen people who visit me don't seem to like too many things hanging on the wall. They unscrew the screws from the wall and let the pictures drop to the floor. Some has to be repaired because the shells broke when they landed on the floor. Other pictures scratched the newly painted walls as they slipped down the wall behind the furniture. To please my unseen friends I have not put them back in case they decide to throw them across the room and break something.

Oh, I need a room to store all my dolls, bears, rabbits and many other stuffed animals which I have made, won, or were given plus all the other keep sakes I have gathered over the years. Presents sent to me from my pen friends. Teaspoon which I have been collecting for years from different towns. Probably a lot of other things which are stored away and I have forgotten are there. One of my prized possessions is a six inch nail which is beginning to rust. This nail was bent in the bare hands of a past friend of the family. It was his party trick to show how strong he was.

I nearly forgot one of the most important rooms in the house, the laundry. In the laundry there would be a few washing machines, wash tubs, dryers, and place for a couple of ironing boards, racks to hang the ironed clothes ready to be wheeled back to the right rooms. Other trolleys to pile all the other clothes and linen on to be taken back to the

Ruth Macklin

cupboards to be put away.

Out in the front of the castle would be a fountain. The driveway would circle around the fountain to drive down the other side of the driveway which would then take you from the front of the castle. In the middle of the both roads would be a row of shrubs all the way to the gates with gardens on outer side of the driveway. The road would be paved to try to minimise the dust in the times when no rain fell to keep the plants, and lawn alive, to help stop the dust from blowing into the castle.

In the grounds at the back of the house would be a small lake with an island in the middle. There would be a bridge for people to walk over to the garden area where there would be a rotunda to sit in away from the boiling sun, a cool shady place to sit and ponder with nature surrounding you. A place to have a picnic in the summer months when looking to find a cool spot. Canoes for those who want to venture around the lake, whether or not, contemplating to encourage their companion romance was in the wind. To try to find a nice cool and private place, so they could be on their own.

Even though I am not a water person I would like to have a swimming pool with a very shallow end. Or my own special swimming pool where my feet touch the bottom and only about waist high. I may have been born under the fish sign but I don't swim like a fish. I sink like a stone if my feet can't touch bottom. I know, because there have been many times where I fell into the water and got out of my depth. Maybe if the teacher had listened to me when I was younger and was being taught to swim in a river, I would have

Ruth Macklin

felt more secure in water and have learnt to swim. But I seem to be getting away from my dreams and back to reality.

At one corner at the side of the pool would be a waterfall where the water goes up through the stones and cascade down over them back into the pool. It would be filtered as it was pumped up the inside of the structure and return over the rocks to look like a waterfall. There would be a small area where people could sit under the fall of the water as it sprayed back towards the pool. Also have a diving board for those who were game enough to dive into the water or want to dive in to show off to impress someone, if they so desired.

But me I would prefer to stay in the smaller pool where I could laze in the cool water to keep cool on the boiling hot days. Or better still, have another pool which was closed in so it could be used in the Summer without being burnt, of freeze during the colder months of winter. I burn easily so it looks as though there will have to be an indoor pool in the dream. Maybe there could be a steam room in the same enclosure to help cleanse away the worry and tiredness, aches and pains, from the body to keep it healthy.

There would be a vegetable and herb gardens to supply the castle with food which would be fresh, not covered with chemicals to keep them or make them grow faster. I would also like to grow a lot of different berries, such as raspberries, blueberries, blackberries, strawberries. Banana plants and citrus trees, custard apples and mangoes would be planted through out the property.

Ruth Macklin

A stable for some horses with a small paddock for them to graze, where anyone could go for a ride if they so desired. I used to have a couple of horses but had to sell them when I moved from the country back to the city for health problems. Looking after the few acres became too much to do on my own when I had to have a few operations. The arthritis wouldn't let me do much heavy work. If I were to accomplish my dreams I would not have to do all the work on my own. I could employ some people to do all the work. So I have to try to work out a way to accomplish all the things of my dream and at the same time be able to bring joy to some other people along the way.

In another part of the garden there would be a chapel for anyone who would like to be married at the Castle of Angels. A place to go for those who would like to pray to what ever God they wanted to talk to, or pray to the Angels, or just a place where they could find some peace in their own life. A place to go to find guidance and harmony in their future life.

I would also like a place in the garden where I could commune with the Celestial forces and the Angels, as well as a place to make my spells if I feel I need some extra help along the way to keep good karma in my future life. A place open to the sun, moon and the stars which would twinkle brightly over the country side. But first I have to completely rid my body of all the bad, suffocating, stressful karma which has been dogging my life for many years. It is time I stood up to fight to get rid of those troubles and not sit back and cry woe is me!waiting for it to pass me by. To leave me free to live a better, calmer life.

Ruth Macklin

I know there are a lot of psychic people, and Celestial forces, who have been edging

me on to free myself, to help me along the way to freedom. I hear from them by snail

mail, e-mail, and come floating through the air to show me they are all there championing

me on to succeed. For me to have a brighter life. So I can help them carry on the good

work they have been doing for years without being acknowledged for countless number

of centuries. Trying to help the people of the world without a thank you because there

were many who do not believe there is any other body to pray to except their one and only

God. They close their mind to what could be a better world if all the killing stopped. All

this senseless slaughter, and killings, because one group of people think their God, or

what ever they call him, were more important than the one the others worship. Those who

try to make others conform to their God by force is not a God worthy of the name.

A God who has to have house bought and paid for by the people who worship him is a

selfish God. You don't really need elaborate buildings with gold trimmings to pray. All

you need to do is pray where ever you feel comfortable. You don't have to put a label on

your faith as everyone has their own opinions. Or should have their own opinions on

where they pray and in who they wish to pray to for help to save their souls. Today? way

of thinking has been clouding our minds so that we can't see what could be out there in

the universe. The churches are trying to keep us hidden under a giant cloud and not allow

us to think for our selves. It is a process which has been clouding the way of thinking for

thousands of years by a few who think they know what is the best for the rest of the

Ruth Macklin

people. Its time to make a change for the betterment of all mankind and let go of the strangle hold a few have who think they know what would be best for all the people of this dying world. A world which has been falling to pieces because there have been too many bombs, and other explosions. The bombs are putting the world out of balance. Causing nature to wreck havoc on mankind. Now is the time to act to reclaim the world from the few and give peace back to every living person, and creature. Bring everlasting peace to the world before there is no world left to live in.

Ruth Macklin

Chapter Two

Water! It is something, which we cannot do without. As I was born under the water sign you would think I would think I'd be able by nature of the sign, to swim like a fish. But I'm not very fond of water. Water is for drinking and bathing but put me near a larger body of water and I'm lost. Maybe it has been all the thing, which have happened to me near a body of water. Being baptised I think was the start of me being afraid of water. The water may have been trickled over my forehead but to me it was like having my head dunked under the water, which had been stored in a drum. This idea had stuck in my memory for years buried deep in my subconscious, which surfaces from time to time. Especially when water is splashed on my face taking away my breath.

Or it could come from all the times I have fallen into the water where I couldn't touch the ground with my feet. Maybe it was all the times I was in the car when my father drove us across flooded creeks to get to where we were going. It seemed as though there was always someone there to guide us through all the large bodies of water. Not always someone of human body. Or maybe it was the years of practice when my father was younger which enabled us to get through the flood water to get to the nearest town for some food.

One of the next occasions where water was involved I was only a few years old. We

Ruth Macklin

lived out in the country where we had to live in a tent made of pieces of tarpaulin. There were poles buried in the ground to hold up the tarpaulin with a pole across the middle at the top which the tarpaulins were thrown over. There were poles which run along either side at a lower level as an anchored for the roof. Then were smaller pieces of tarpaulin wrapped around the poles to make walls. A piece across the middle in side to make a bedroom and kitchen area. Wooden pallets were placed on the ground to make flooring inside the tent before beds and other furniture were placed inside to make it feel like a home.

At the kitchen end of the tent a corrugated iron stove recess was built to house a wood stove to do the cooking. For a shower we had a frame built of wood with corrugated iron around three side and with a wooden door. There was no roof to the shower room. A single board was bolted across the top from which hung an iron bucket to be filled with water. The water would be released when the string attached to a liver was pulled to to open the holes to let the water flow through. Very cold in the winter months which meant you had quick showers before you became cold, or you turned blue. In the winter we would run into the tent to stand in front of the blazing hot fire in the stove to get warm. You also had to watch you didn't have unwanted guests in the shower with you, things like frogs, toads, or snakes. They would appear from under the pallet when the water began to flow.

In the wet weather when it used to rain a lot, we were forced to bath in a small round

Ruth Macklin

tin tub which was placed on the floor in front of the stove in the kitchen. Each of us had to get in the tub one after the other with the cleanest people to have a bath first. Most of the time dodging the washing which hung near the stove to dry. In those days when you had to boil your clothes in coppers in the dry weather, or in a four gallon kerosene tin on the stove, when it was pouring rain. There were no washing machines, dryers, or electricity, which is available today for an easier life. Lights were kerosene lanterns or carbine lights.

When we were living there mum got very sick and she kept telling us she could see Angels flying around inside the tent. She said they were so pretty with their long white dresses with flowers twisted in their long hair. Their big wings fluttering as they hovered over the bottom of her bed. It was one of those times when the creeks came up over night and there was no way to get to the nearest town. She was seeing the Angels for a few day until the worse of the sickness past and she started to regain her health.

In the days of long ago when you knew you could depend on the rain to fall when it should the rain always came on time to help those who needed it. The farmers didn't have to worry about when the rain would fall. The fall of heavy rain kept the rivers clean and flowing. The grass kept its beautiful green colour most of the time so there was plenty of food for the animals.

The trees were all different shades of green to show their good health. People didn't moan everyday about the weather. The strong winds did not blow the fertile top soil away

Ruth Macklin

into the ocean and leave the ground a barren waste land. You only had to pee up in the

top region of the rivers and they would be in flood for days. The rain did not have to fall

in you area but the creeks would be running a banker and the sun would be shining

brightly in the blue sky above your head.

One such week it rained buckets with no sign of the rain stopping. The rivers were

rising fast making it impossible for people to move through the area. Fresh food supplies

had become very low. The trains were the only way to bring fresh supplies in to you if

you could get someone to send them to you. Or you had to catch the rail motor to the

closest large town which was Bundaberg some fifty miles away. You would have to catch

the early morning rail motor and return late at night lugging your bags of food. You never

knew when the flood waters would subside enough for a car to be able to cross the low

crossings to be able to get to town to do your shopping. You always had to have an extra

supply of tin food to carry you over in the times when the rivers were impassable.

Sometimes you could not be prepared for the flood as it would come without much

warning. The rain would sneak in during the cover of the night soaking the ground and

making it muddy by morning. On one such occasion the rain fell heavy during the night

and the river near where we lived rose fast causing trouble for the gang of bridge workers.

The gang were there to replace the old wooden piles of the bridge with cement ones. The

men were pulled out of bed to go down to the creek to rescue all the tools which would

soon be washed down the creek if they were not moved to higher ground.

Ruth Macklin

As the men struggled in the rain, mud and water, to try to move everything a roar could be heard as the wall of water rushed down the creek pushing all the rubbish and dead timber with the water on its escape to the bigger river to reach the ocean. The wheels of the cement mixers began bogging in the mud making it ten times as hard as the men struggle to get the machinery to safety. Bags of cement were moved from the shed and taken to an empty hut where the men were camped.

Everything was wet and there was no sign of the rain letting up. We were surrounded by flood water in all directions. Food was becoming less as the days passed. People were trying to make their food go further and not waste any. Opening tins of food because there was not much fresh food left. No one knew when they would be able to leave their work to go to town to get some fresh supplies.

Our tent was wet through. Our clothes smelt musty. Felt damp. The clothes could not be washed because there was no where to hang them except inside the tent in front of the stove to get them dry. A rope line had to be strung across the front of the stove recess to peg the clothes on to dry. The wood stove had to be kept going to try to air out the tent and cook the food. Some clothes were also hung over the backs of the chairs which were placed close to the wood stove when it was not in use for cooking meals. We had to keep ducking our head so we would not become hung on the line ourself.

During this latest bout of wet weather the kerosene which was used to keep the fridges began running out. The wick which soaked up the kerosene was turned back to save on

Ruth Macklin

kerosene and keep the fridges working longer. Hoping this would keep food cold until the
sun began to shine once more.

On one busy day Jack had not take the meat out of the tin he had just opened. In his
rush to get back to work he had left it sitting on the table. Even though it was raining the
weather was still muggy. A combination of meat left in a tin and hot weather was a sure
sign of trouble. Worse possible solution in the 1950's when tins were tin. The food was
not given a thought when the men rushed back to work to watch the railway bridge did
not wash away with the flood waters. The open tin had been left forgotten on the table
until Jack returned back to camp later in the afternoon for his evening meal. Thinking
because the weather was wet and cool in the hut the food would be still good to eat. Jack
Clarke decided to eat the Bully Beef which had sat in the open tin all afternoon. He
should have known not to eat the meat. Even though the food supplies were getting low.

In the early hours of the next morning Jack began moaning from the pains in his
stomach before the vomiting and the gastric caused him to become very weak. Jack had
gotten wet from rushing backward and forward to the out side toilet. When his legs would
not carry him any more he carried a bucket back in side of the hut in which to be sick.
The other man sharing the hut, Fred Williams, did not get much sleep because of Jack and
his moaning, and being sick. Fred climbed from his bed and went to check on Jack.

Placing his hand on Jack's forehead he found it very hot and wet with perspiration.

Putting on his raincoat Fred headed out to find the boss of the bridge gang to tell him

Ruth Macklin

Jack had taken ill during the night. Fred found his boss standing on the railway bridge watching the rubbish in the water did not build up around the pylons to wash away the bridge. If the bridge had washed away the main railway line to the north and south of the town would stop all rail traffic until the bridge could be re-built.

Fred explained the condition of Jack to Colin Speil, his boss, then Colin went with Fred back to the camp to see Jack for himself. To see if he could find out what was happening to Jack. Colin could not afford his men getting sick as there was no way he would be able to get any of them away to see a doctor. After checking out Jack, Colin decided to ring the hospital in Bundaberg to see what they could suggest could be done to help Fred get better.

Going on what Colin had to tell the doctor the doctor believed Jack was suffering from an appendix attack and he should be taken to the hospital as soon as possible in case Jack needed surgery. Jack would be in big trouble if the problem was his appendix as the appendix could burst. He could die. So it had become dire Jack should be taken in to the hospital as fast as they could.

"You have to be asking me to get Jack to the moon,replied Colin.

"Why?the doctor wanted to know.

Colin went on to explain they were flood bound and there was no way any one could drive Jack to the hospital. It would take too long to send Jack down by rail motor as it had already gone past for the day. Colin told the doctor he would see what he could arrange

Ruth Macklin

and ring him back. Colin had his fingers crossed there would be someone around who would know how he was going to get Jack to the hospital. He would talk to all the men to see if they knew of another way to get Jack across the flooded rivers, and gullies, and low lying flats where the water run down from the hills to rush across the roads.

The men who were not watching the rising water stood waiting at the hut to see how Jack was going to get to the hospital. Some of the men were trying to keep Jack as calm as possible. One washed Jack's forehead with cold water to try to get his temperature to come down. Jack was drenched from the rain and perspiration from his high temperature. The men could see Jack was getting sicker by the minute, his moaning getting louder. His stomach was so empty he was dry retching. The men gathered around the boss to hear what could be done for their mate.

Colin raked his hand through his wet hair. He was hedging on how he was to tell the men there was no way any help would be going to get through to them until all the flood waters began to subside. The stress and the wet weather had started to take a toll on him. They were in a big pickle. There did not seem to be a way of getting help which Colin could see at the moment.

"Well? What did the doctor suggest for us to do?" asked one of the men.

"There is not much we can do," Colin replied, hunching his shoulders. Most of the rivers, creeks and gullies are flooded between here and the hospital in Bundaberg. The ambulance can only make it as far as Smith's Crossing."

Ruth Macklin

"What did the doctor suggest we should do to make Jack feel better?" asked another.

"Told me to find a way to get him to the hospital. The doctor thinks he may have an appendix problem and might need an operation," sighed Colin. "I have no idea how we are going to get Jack out of here to the hospital."

"May be Bert could help. Why don't you ask him if it is possible to get over the creeks to the hospital?" suggested another man. "He has local knowledge of the area."

Colin went down to the bridge to find Bert, my father, to see what he might suggest could be done to get Jack to the hospital. My father listened to what Colin had to say then he made some suggestions on how they might be able to get Jack to the hospital. What would be needed to help my father complete the mission. The idea was discussed with all the other men and soon the plan was being put into action. Colin went back to the railway station to phone the hospital of an attempt being made to get Jack as far as Smith's Crossing. The ambulance could be there to meet them and ferry the patient to the other side of the water.

My father went home to tell mum, Elsa, he was going to have to make a trip to try to get to Bundaberg as one of his work mates were sick. Jack had to be taken to the hospital. Mum was not too pleased with the idea as she could see all the flaws of the best laid plan. She told dad he was bloody stupid to even try to make it as far as Smith's Crossing. There would be too many places where the water would be rushing across the road. She explained some of the bridges could have been washed away but dad could not to be

Ruth Macklin

deterred from his mission. Mum dressed me in a rain coat then grabbed a few dry clothes

for us and put them in a waterproof bag so we would have some dry clothes if we made it

through without being drowned. Soon we were on our way from the tent to the railway

line where a flat top had been hooked behind the pumper to take us across the bridge.

The pumper stopped at the camp site for the men to collect Jack. Some of the men

carried Jack from the hut and loaded him on to the flat top with a small piece of tarpaulin

over him to try to keep him as dry as possible. The men got on the pumper and soon we

were travelling along the railway line to cross the bridge to the other side of the creek

where my father had left his car. He had left it at the home of a friend on the other side of

the creek as we could not get across the creek a couple of weeks ago when we arrived

home from Bundaberg.

My father went to his friend's house to get his car while the men were to carry Jack

down the bank from the railway line. The men helped mum and I to slither down the

muddy bank, through the fence to wait for the car. We were to make the trip with dad and

Jack because mum knew the area. She had lived there when she was a child and knew the

area better than dad did. She might also be needed to drive the car if the car had become

stuck somewhere along the muddy, water logged road, which was an excuse for a road. It

was a little more than a bush track which had been carved out for the people to reach their

homes in the country. It hadn't improved much since the road was first used to drive

sulkies and drays along the road in the days of long ago. The road design gave the

Ruth Macklin

impression that the person who had made the road was drunk, or he had followed a snake. The road was full of twists and turns, up hills and down into gullies. One hump in the road left your stomach up in the air as the car passed down the other side like a roller coaster ride.

The men soon had Jack loaded on to the back seat of the car and we headed off into the unknown not knowing if we would make it to where we were suppose to meet the ambulance. The work men who were allowed to be relieved of their bridge watching duties hopped on the pumper to follow along the railway line beside the road to the end of the section of line to make sure we made our way that far. The fettles gang of the next section came out from Rosedale to make sure we made it to Rosedale. From there we would be on our own as the road swung away from beside the railway line.

The dirt road up the first hill was slippery. The clay was now showing as the surface gravel was partially washed away. My father struggled hard to keep the car wheels on what was left of the gravel as the car slew from side to side to get to the rise of the hill. From there the road was full of ruts where the flood waters flowed across, or along, the road. Dad had to drive with caution through the water which had backed up over sections of the road. The next tough section would be a nightmare. There was a cement causeway which was covered with run-off water flowing across the road with a very steep, red soil hill to travel up once the car had made it through the water.

Dad stopped the car short of the water then went to walk through the water to the other

Ruth Macklin

side to check the crossing for a washout, or rocks, or any other stuff which may hamper the car making its way through the water. He then walked up the hill stamping his feet to find out where the ground was soft, and hard. By the time the road had been checked the workmen had arrived on the pumper. The pumper was pulled off the line to sit on the siding in case there was a train coming along that section of line. The workmen slid their way down the steep embankment and climbed through the fence to reach the road.

Ruth Macklin

Chapter Three

There were a few minutes of discussion on the best way to approach the crossing. How to drive through the water and up the slippery hill. A couple of workmen searched around to find a few pieces of dead wood, or stones, to use as chocks to hold the car from slipping all the way back down the hill into the water. All the workmen made their way to the other side of the water and part way up the hill to wait for my father to drive his car slowly through the water, because going fast would have wet the spark plug wires and we would have been stuck there until the wires had dried out. Too much speed would also carry too much water up on to the already saturated mud making the driving of the car worse.

Mum and I had been made get out of the car to walk through the water and make our own way up the hill to wait for the car to get there. No one could predict what might have happened if the car had gotten out of control. The car could have crashed into the bank at the side of the road. Or rolled if it had slipped the wrong way. There was a lot of danger to everyone concerned on that struggle against nature. No one was hurt in the struggle but they were covered in mud from head to boots.

The drive through the water was very slow. As soon as the front wheels had come out of the water my father put his foot down heavy on the accelerator to get some much needed speed to get as far as he could before the wheel began to spin in the mud. The

men were ready with the chocks to put under the wheels as well as try to keep out of the

way so they would not get run over as the car spun from side to side. My father had to

hang on tight to the steering wheel to keep control of the car so it would not swing right

around and face back down the hill. Some men tried to stop the car sliding backward as

others placed the chocks. Their shoes slipping in the mud with not much traction. Then

some would try to push the car to help it get more traction to get a little further up the hill

before it had to be chocked again. The men worked in this manner until the car reached

the top of the hill where the ground was a bit firmer. My father and the men finally got

the car to the top without anyone getting hurt. That was Royal's Gully crossed. We were

now travelling into the unknown without any idea how much further we would be able to

go. How much water there would be to stop us reaching our destination.

One of the workmen got elected to go in the car with us for back up as the men could

see that my father would not be able to handle it all on his own if there were any more

problems ahead. Sam Conway got in the back of the car with Jack and we continued on

with our journey to the hospital. The rest of the workmen took the pumper back to

Berajondo to wait for news. The fettler gang watched our progress as the car made its way

to Rosedale. The Rosedale gang were to let the other know we had passed through

the small town. Once we had passed through the town we were on our own for the rest of

the trip. The road snaked away from the train line so there was no way we could be

Ruth Macklin

followed. People were asked to watch as we crossed railway crossings to see how far we had made it.

Bottle Creek and some of the other gullies were flowing across the road. At each body of flowing water my father got out of the car to check the crossing to see if there were no wash out or rubbish on the road. Doing this for safety our progress was very slow. We travelled as safely as was possible in the bad weather. During the drive there were showers of rain which made it hard to see if any trees had been blown over the road. Otherwise the trees would have had to be removed because there would have been no chance of getting off the narrow, unsealed road. Having to stop to cut a tree from across the road would have taken more time of which we didn't have. Some small branches had to be shifted off the road but nothing too heavy.

Most of the trip went well, but slow, until the place which was to be our biggest worry, Smith's Crossing. It was a creek which would flood quickly if someone did a pee in the creek. It was a spooky place in the sunny weather but was more frightening in the dark. A place where a criminal, or someone wishing a good place to murder someone and hide the body in the scrub up so close to the side of the road. Everyone was of the opinion the ambulance would be there waiting on the other side of the flood water with a boat to ferry Jack across the large body of swiftly flowing brown flood water. On reaching the bottom of the hill there was only a few feet of reasonably dry ground between the now stationary car and the savage body of brown flood water. There was no sign of the

Ruth Macklin

ambulance car, or ambulance men, or any one with a boat to help Jack across the water to be taken to the hospital.

After about half an hour wait, two ambulance men walked down the small hill on the other side, crossing the little wooden bridge over the gully full with back water which lapped just beneath the decking to make their way to the edge of the water. My father yelled to them and the ambulance man yelled back but no one seemed to be able to hear what the other one had to say. So my father started to make his way through the water to the other side keeping to the right side of the causeway so he would not be swept off the edge without a hope of being saved. He watched there were no logs, or branches, floating down with the flood water. He finally made it to the other side to find out what was to happen. After a long discussion about how to get Jack to the other side, and his health at the moment, my father made his way back through the water to us waiting in the car.

"What are they going to do?" My Mother asked, with worry etched on her face. She knew something was not right because she could see the ambulance men shaking their heads in disbelief. "You're not going to try to cross that?" My Mother's voice rising with the thought of us crossing that very wide section of rushing, and swirling water. "We'll all be drowned when the car was washed off the causeway. There was not a chance we would make it across to the other side alive."

"That's the only way to go. There's no other help coming" .My father got the key out of the ignition then he went to open the boot of the car where he pulled out the thick piece of tarpaulin, which the men used to sit under to have their lunch. Along with a

Ruth Macklin

couple of spanners from the tool box. My father then lifted the bonnet and began working

on taking off the fan-belt so it would not churn up water to wet the spark plugs, or any

other part which would stall the engine. All special parts were covered with old oil rags to

keep the parts dry for as long as possible to get us to the other side of the water. Next the

piece of tarpaulin was placed over the front of the car once the bonnet had been closed to

keep more water away from the engine. The tarpaulin had to be tied to the bumper bar at

the front and the doors of the car so the tarpaulin would not wash off once the car entered

the water. The driver's side headlight was left out to show where we were headed. Sam

sat on the mudguard as a guide. He also had to hold the tarpaulin in place and watch for

any rubbish coming down with the flood waters. The ambulance men stood as guides to

show where the edge of the causeway started and ended.

Jack was propped up against the car door with packing put beside him to make sure he

did not slip back down on to the seat because the water was going to come into the car.

The water looked as though it would reach half way up the side of our car. We were all

praying nothing would go wrong in the middle as there would have been no chance of any

of us surviving as most of us could not swim to save our lives. I had no hope at the age of

three years. If the car got washed off the causeway there would have been no hope of

trying as the car would have been battered against the trees hidden in the water.

My father started the engine of the car. He began to slowly edge the front of the car

into the water. I hung on tightly to the back of the front seat where I was standing. We

Ruth Macklin

made it on to the first little wooden bridge with the guide posts showing the edge. The

water began to seep into the car. The car began to edge sideways once we got on to the

cement section of the causeway. The car felt as though it were about to float.

"Open you bloody door to let the water out,yelled my father to my mother.

My Mother opened the door on her side of the car and the car settled on a straight path

once again. Nearing the other side there was a slight dip in the cement and the water

became deeper but not rushing as hard. The water in the car was touching the bottom of

the steering wheel. Six feet from making our way safely to the other side and up the small

rise where we would be able to stop the car to transfer Jack to the ambulance, the engine

spluttered and died.

"Get out of the bloody car and push!yelled my Father, as he forced his door open to be

able to get out to push and steer the car out of the water.

Sam Conway jumped off the mudguard and made his way through the water to the

back of the car to help push. Both of the ambulance men plunged into the water to help

push, and push, as it was very hard with the car full of water but we won out in the end.

My Mother collapsed on to the seat of the car as her shaking legs would not hold her up

any more. I hung on the the back of the seat with water dripping from my clothes. My

fingers didn't seem to want to let go.

The ambulance men open the back door of the car to check Jack who had been

unaware of what had just happened. Jack was soon transferred to the back of the

Ruth Macklin

ambulance to be taken to the hospital. "You are not going back across that water?" asked one of the ambulance men.

"No," replied my Father. "Once I get the engine dried out and going we will continue on into Bundaberg."

"Do you want us to send someone to help you get the car started?"

"We'll be fine,my father said, going to fetch his tools out of the boot of the car.

When we arrived at our destination, got dried, we rang the hospital to find out what the doctor had found wrong with Jack. We were told Jack was going to get better. He was suffering from a very bad case of food poisoning. Jack would be in the hospital for a couple of weeks. The return trip home was a lot better and dry. We took the rail motor back to Berajondo the next afternoon. The sun had once again come out to dry up some of the excess water. Dry our wet clothes. To soak up some of the water left behind. To wait until the water had flowed away to open the road until the next time the heavens opened to cause more floods.

On another occasion when there was sign of rain to come bucketing down we had raced into Bundaberg to stock up with food but in the rush care was not taken. The boot was full with food and the back seat with a little, tiny space, left on the back seat for me. I got in the car and pulled the door shut. I was squashed between the bags of food and the door. We set out for home. Drove through the streets and over the Burnett traffic bridge and turned left once on the other side. As my father followed the curve in the road there

Ruth Macklin

came a whoosh of air from the back of the car. My mother turned her head to see what the

noise was. To her horror I was not seated on the back seat. I was gone. When the latch on

the door, which must not have clicked properly, let go I rolled out of the car door. Lucky

for me there were no cars coming on to the bridge from the other side. Or a train was

using the train line. No bones were broken. But I had bandages on my arms and legs for

weeks. I was sore all over. It was painful for me to walk. After that my parents made sure

I was in the middle of the seat and both doors locked. If the door did come open again

only food would fall out which could easily be replaced. The doctors said I was very

lucky not to have any bones broken. We still made it home before the creeks had a chance

to flood.

Then there was another time when the wet had arrived and decided to stay for awhile. I

have not forgotten this one. It was a hard lesson on what not to do on a wet, boring week.

The wooden stove was roaring hot. Washing had been strung around the kitchen in the

tent. My mother was making cakes and scones for my father when he came home for

smoko. I was bored because I could not go out side to play. Boredom usually turns to

trouble. Which I sorely found out.

My mother had her back to me while mixing up the dough for the scones. I sat on the

floor complaining there was nothing for me to do. My mother gave me a very simple job

to do for her. I had to find a couple of baking trays in the cupboard. An old wooden

cupboard with a few shelves on which stood the dinner set, glasses, baking dishes of all shapes and sizes, glass mixing bowels. It was all packed in neatly. It should have been heavy and hard to shift. As I found out the cupboard was easy to shift.

Because I was taking so long to produce the cake trays my mother turned to see what was taking me so long. I had just put my full weight on one of the open doors. "Don't swing on...." was as far as my mother got before there came loud breaking, and banging, noises when the cupboard tipped to empty all the contents on the floor.

All the tin dished banged and clattered around the floor. Most of the glass and china lay in bits, and pieces on the floor. In one way I was lucky. The door I had been swinging on stopped the cupboard from completely falling over on to the floor. After much shouting my mother produced a four gallon kerosene tin for me to pick up the pieces. It was the only way I could get out from standing in the middle of all the broken glassware. The tin was nearly full when I had finished picking up all the pieces. Once the floor around me had been swept it was time for my punishment. The wooden baking spoon was smacked across my backside and I was sent to bed.

Later when my father came in from being out in the rain at work the first thing he spotted was the tin of broken glassware. When he had been told what happened, I nearly got a second lot of punishment from him but my mother said she had already given me my punishment and sent to bed without getting any of the hot scones. I knew not to swing on that cupboard door ever again. After that day tin plates were produced to eat on as we travelled around a lot.

Ruth Macklin

Some where along on our travels we ended up in Rockhampton where my parents took up cutting timber for a living. We cut short lengths of timber which were taken from the scrub to the nearest railway siding, where the timber would be loaded on to train wagons to be transported to the mill to be sawn into sleepers. These wooden sleepers were used before the invention of the cement sleepers which are used today. The finding of the right trees to cut down was very hard work. Even harder to get them out of the scrub.

Each morning before the sun rose to bring in the new day we were out of bed and had our breakfast. Lunch made to take with so we would not have to return to the camp until the truck had been loaded to take to be delivered to the railway yard. The chainsaw chain had been sharpened before we went to bed even if the time was late. Water bottles filled. Fuel and oil put on the truck to last the day. As the sun rose high enough for my father to see where he was driving we set off into the bush from the open sided shed where we slept. Well where my parents slept. I had to sleep on the back seat of the car. In the shed was an old double bed for them to sleep on. There was an old wooden stove on which to cook our food and not much else.

All day we would push our way through the bush looking for the right trees. My mother and I would follow behind with the heavy tools which would be needed to do the job. My father would walk around the base of the tree looking upward to see if it was straight enough for cutting, no knobs, which meant he would loose some of the tree if he was to cut that tree. The real straight, tall trees were cut down and saved to take to the

Ruth Macklin

sawmill to be cut into timber for building houses. The left overs would be used for sleepers.

The truck would be left a fair distance so no trees would fall on the truck. My mother and I would have to stand back from the tree in case the wind blew while the tree was being cut and the tree fell in the wrong direction. Some times my mother would have to go to stand next to my father to hammer wedges into the cut of the tree because the blade of the chainsaw had become stuck and my father could not pull it out. You had to be quick of foot once the tree began to fall so you would not be crushed beneath and killed. Thankfully someone was watching over us and we never got hurt by a falling tree.

Once the tree lay on the ground it had to be cut up into blocks. My father had a light piece of wood cut to the right length of a sleeper block which either my mother or I, laid it along the fallen tree to show my father where he had to saw. My mother had to stand close to where my father was sawing the log with a hammer and wedge, to hammer the wedge into the top of the cut to keep the cut open and not jam the saw blade. Some times it was very hard for her to see with the saw dust flying in the air. They would both be covered with saw dust. When the sawing had been finished it came time to remove the bark from the sleeper blocks but not from the pieces which were to go to the timber mill. Sometimes the removal of the bark was easy. Other times it was real hard. Especially on some of the trees at certain times of the year.

My father would chop across the top of the log with the axe then the crowbar dug

Ruth Macklin

under the bark to remove it. You had to be careful tools didn't slip when the bark gave

away. Sometimes we had to hold the log with a special kind of hook to keep it in place

while dad worked to get off the bark. When the bark was removed there was another

danger of which you had to be careful. If you stood on the inside of the bark which was

wet you found you were soon sitting down heavily on the ground, or the bark, even if you

wore rubber soled shoes.

Ruth Macklin

Chapter Four

Once the tray of the truck was loaded we wended our way through the scrub to find our way to the road on which we'd travel to take the load to the railway storage yard to unload the sleeper blocks. When the wire rope had been taken away from over the load, the stays at the back of the tray were belted hard with a fourteen pound hammer in an upward direction then all the blocks fell to the ground. My father had to be quick of foot to get out of the way once the second stay had been knocked out. If my father hadn't moved out of the way quickly he would have been injured, or killed, as large blocks rolled on to the ground. Thankfully, that never happened. My father made sure we were all out of harms way. When the last block had been rolled off of the tray to the stack, we would get back into the truck and head back out to the scrub to cut another load of blocks to take to the railway yard just as the sun was on it's way to bed.

Day after day, we worked like slaves until Friday afternoon when we would load the truck with long logs of timber to take to the sawmill for the timber to be sawn into different sizes for the use of building houses. The loads were heavy and hung over the back of the truck by two, or three feet.

"That is enough. The truck won't pull the load if you put any more on". My mother was always telling my father, but he just went on his merry way and loaded the extra log, or two, on the top of the load. He was trying to save on trips because the time taken to deliver small loads would cut in to his working hours. One bigger load was his way to go.

"Of course I can. There's plenty of room for another one. He would have a look under the side of the truck to see how far the tyres were from the tray of the truck. "Still enough wheel room to take another." So away he went to and snug the next log to the truck with the tractor to be loaded.

My mother and I would shake our heads in disbelief. There was no point in arguing about the out come because what my father decided was law, the law on the timber master. Once the next log had been put in place the load had to be secured with chains to stop the load moving. Or falling off the truck on to some cars as we drove along the highway to Rockhampton to get to the sawmill. I still shake my head to think the truck made its way slowly up all those big hills. I would have been complaining if I would have

had to carry such a heavy load but the engine didn't miss a beat. Most times I don't know how my father could steer the truck because there was more weight at the back of the truck than the front. The tyres were just touching the road. Most time I felt the road was lifting to touch the tyres. Or there were a few Guardian Angels travelling with us to keep the truck on the road.

One night I thought we were goners. We had to follow a track to reach the sawmill yard which swung around a sharp curve on to a small wooden bridge across a gully to reach the place to dump the logs. We were late leaving the paddock then had to fight our way through Friday night traffic. The sun had dropped below the horizon by the time we

Ruth Macklin

reached the entrance to the sawmill yard. My father had to have his one more log. We were crawling along at a steady pace as we came to the curve. The weight on the back of the truck made it hard on the brakes. The weight of the timber on the back of the truck pushed forward as we went down the slight slope to the bridge.

"We're not going to make it,my mother complained, seeing us crushed to our deaths in the gully with the load of logs on top of us.

"Of course we'll make it. My father was so sure, or pretended he was not scared. Positive he would make the bridge, or die trying. Fate would not dare to disagree with him.

I kept my eyes focused on the lights of the sawmill because they would have been the last thing I would have seen. I didn't want to look at that narrow bridge. It's a wonder the weight of the truck never broke through the wooden bridge. The front of the truck seemed to turn in the right direction to line up with the narrow bridge to take the truck through to the yard. The weight must have put the tyers on the ground enough for my father to be able to steer the truck across the bridge.

"I told you we would make it,is all my Father would say when we were safely across the bridge and headed to dump the load.

"You stupid idiot! You could have killed us all. You were lucky the truck knew where to go. Next time you want to put on one more you deliver it on your own.?ut next time we were there even with the one extra log on the top of the load.

Ruth Macklin

On one occasion when we were sleeping at the shed, me on the back seat of the car where I usually slept. My mother and my father on the bed in the open sided shed. My mother had a feeling they were not the only ones in the bed. There was nothing wrong with the bed when they had gotten in to go to sleep. Ten minutes later they were joined by an unwelcome visitor.

"Turn on the car lights,my father yelled to me. It was quicker than trying to light a pressure light. Or find a torch.

I crawled over the back of the front seat to get to the light switch. Searched in the dark for the light switch to turn on the car headlights. Then there came a scream from my mother as she scrambled out of the bed to run for the car to get in side and shut the door. I looked toward the bed to see what had happened. There, slithering across the bottom of the bed was a very large Carpet snake out in search for his food. In the shed mice lived among the cattle food stored in the other section of the shed. He was just taking a short cut to find his food.

That was the end of my mother sleeping in the bed, or the shed. She spent the rest of the night sitting in the front of the car sleeping. The snake was the last straw. This way of life no longer appealed to her. She wanted out. My father had to find another way to earn money for us to live. Or a different place to sleep. A few weeks later my father was offered another job of working for the railway again. A caravan was bought so we would be able to follow the gang as the gang moved from place to place. My father kept putting

Ruth Macklin

in for different jobs until we finally ended up back at Berajondo.

The caravan was backed in under a very large Jacaranda Tree. Holes were dug to put

posts in to hold up a couple of tarpaulins to shade the caravan and protect it from the

flowers and leaves falling from the tree. Wooden pallets were laid along one side of the

caravan to be used as a kitchen. A corrugated iron stove recess had to be built at the back

end in which was placed a wooden stove. A long wooden bench was placed on the pallet

floor to use for cooking, and washing the dishes. A kerosene fridge was added to keep the

food in as the one in the caravan was too small. The car went under the front part of the

tent and the good old truck was parked there in front of our new home. A large tank was

set up on some pallets to hold water for drinking, and everything else. The train would

bring water through every week for all of us to fill our tanks.

Once more we had our out door shower. The one made of corrugated iron, wooden

pallet for the floor and no roof. This time we had to share the shower with the man who

lived in the hut next to us. So once again we had to pull the rope to get wet. Wash your

self with the soap and washer then rinse the soap away. Early, quick showers when the

months move into winter. Summer time it was great showering under the stars. Unless it

was raining.

Our washing was done by putting our clothes in an out side copper boiler. The fire had

to be lit early to get the water to boil before it was time to put in the clothes. Wood had to

be added to the fire to keep it burning until the last of the washing was finished. When the water had cooled it had to be bailed out and tipped down over the side of the bank behind

the caravan. A couple of pieces of wire had to be strung between two posts on which

hang our clothes. A wooden prop made from a tree branch with a fork at the top to hold

the wire up to keep the clothes from dragging on the ground. When the prop broke the

washing would end up in the dirt and would have to be washed once again. You had to

keep a few props handy for the times when one did break. You couldn't always have time

to go looking for one if it broke at the wrong time.

The toilet was a thunder box type. There were three walls of corrugated iron for walls

and a piece of tarpaulin hung down the front for the door. A drum had to be placed under

a wooden box with a hole in the top to sit on when using the toilet. You didn't stay too

long as it could become very smelly at times. The worst job came when the drum was

near full. A hole had to be dug in the ground. A crowbar had to be used to dig the ground

to loosen the hard dirt and clay. The loose dirt was then dug out with a shovel. The

process had to be done until the hole was big enough to empty in the smelly contents

from the drum. The idea was to hold the nose with one hand, tip gently and try to keep

out of the way so you did not get splashed then quickly shovel the soil over the top to get

rid of the smell. Not like today when you just have to push a button. And you don't have

to watch for frogs, toads, snakes or spiders. The frogs and toads would hide under the

pallet floor and wait their chance to sneak under the tarpaulin door.

As there were no dumps we had to dig holes to bury our tins and other rubbish. There

Ruth Macklin

seemed to be always something to do with hard work. Chopping firewood was another

hard job especially if my father didn't cut the right dead trees to bring home for firewood.

The chopped wood had to be carried in to the kitchen area and placed in a box near the

wood stove. You had to be careful how you loaded the wood on your arm to carry

otherwise you would have digs, scratches, or splinters.

The guy in the hut on the other side of the caravan didn't have his own toilet so he had

to use the one over at the railway station which the workers used and so did the train

passengers. He had his own corrugated iron stove recess in which he had a wood stove

but not much protection while cooking in wet, and windy weather. There was a roof from

the hut to the recess but it was no protection from the weather.

On one of the big limbs of the Jacaranda tree my father made me a swing with thick

rope and a wooden seat. It was a very cool place to sit in the warmer weather. I remember

sitting there on the swing with two of my father's six inch nails, and some of the bits of

left over wool from my mother to practice how to knit. I would practice the stitch until

the wool ran out then the wool would be slipped off the nails and pulled undone once my

mother had checked to see if the stitch had been done right. I then had to practice the next

stitch. It was very time consuming as there were no other children to play with at the time.

I only ever had one doll which I had to look after because I knew I would not get

another one as money for food was more important. I also had a doll's pram. My mother

made clothes for the doll with scraps of material left over from sewing our clothes. Some

Ruth Macklin

doll's clothes were knitted from scraps of wool. I would sit for hours dressing, and re-dressing, the doll to push it around the caravan, or sit on the swing and push the pram as I slowly swung back and forward.

That is, until I some how received a kitten for my very own. It was a ginger male cat. Ginger became very quiet and I could do almost any thing with him. I could dress Ginger in my doll's dresses. Tie a bonnet on his head. Place him in the doll's pram to pat him to sleep and he would stay there for hours without trying to get out and run away with the clothes still on him. Lots of people were surprised Ginger would allow me to dress him in doll's clothes.

But one fatal day my world fell apart so I thought. I came home from school to find Ginger was not where he usually slept. I called his name but there didn't come an answer. Ginger wandered all around the paddocks and across the other side of the railway lines searching for extra food. This day he was not quick enough.

"Where's Ginger?" asked, after I dropped my school bag in the door of the caravan. "He's not in his usual place."

"I had to get Ginger put to sleep," my Mother told me, but I didn't believe her.

"How could you do that? He was my best friend in the world. Why did you do it?" I yelled, as the tears rolled down my cheeks.

"I had no choice," my Mother told me as she tried to calm me. "Ginger had been run over by a train. He must have been running across the line when the train came through.

Ruth Macklin

He had no legs. It would have been cruel to let him suffer."

I stormed out of the caravan and ran around to my swing to sit there and cry my heart

out for my friend I would never see again. It was just one of those unfortunate facts of

life. Living close to railway lines and busy roads are a hazard to all animals. You never

knew when your best friend would not return to you. It took me a fair while before I

wanted another pet to call my own. Or my best friend! Even though the animals were

more reliable than most of the children at the school. The children were farmers sons and

daughters and were not very kind to new arrivals. Or to any one who didn't belonged to a

family who had lived in the area for a very long time. Even though I was a distant relation

to some I was still not acceptable as a close friend.

Berajondo state School stood on the top of a steep, stony hill. The building was a

small wooden structure with a front verandah. There was only the one room and all

classes were taught by the one teacher. The toilets, or dunnies as they were often called,

were wooden structures set well away from the school building. The water supply came

from two rain water tanks on stands beside the school. The school was the same building

my mother, her sisters and brothers, went to when they had to attend school.

In their time at school they had to walk about five miles to reach the school by cutting

through farmers paddocks. When I went there I had to walk along a gravel track which

was called a road to reach the school. The distance was about a mile from the railway

station. If I were lucky I would get a ride by on of the farmers half way, or dropped in

Ruth Macklin

front of the school on their way past to their farm when it was cream day. Cream day the

farmers brought their cans of cream into the railway station to be loaded on to the train to

be taken to Bundaberg where the cream became butter. That was, when Bundaberg had

their own butter factory which is now gone.

My parents bought a bicycle for me to ride to school but it became a lot safer to walk. I

learnt the hard way not to ride my bicycle down the steep hill. The problem was not that I

couldn't ride slowly down the hill. The main worry for me stood in a line stretched all the

way across the road. The human line! They all spaced themselves across the road so there

was no way to get around them. No one of them would move out of the way. When I had

to put more pressure on the peddles to stop the wheels skidded on the loose gravel and I

landed on the gravel road. I didn't cry! No way was I going to cry! I dusted off my clothes,

legs and arms, picked up the bicycle while they stood there laughing at me. I walked the

rest of the way down the hill before I got back on the bicycle to ride the rest of the way

home. My Mother wanted to know how I came to get all the scratches.

The wheels skidded on the gravel. I'll be walking down the hill in future. If I was quick

out to my bicycle and on the road first I road down the hill but otherwise I walked down

the school hill.

The children who played their game of chicken on me were not the only danger which

lurked along the road. On one section of the road there was another attacker during

nesting season. The Magpies! As any one rode by the Magpies would swoop down to

Ruth Macklin

pick you on the head. I got picked on the top of the head once. From then on I walked past the area where the Magpies nested up in the trees. Kept a hat on my head when I realised it was time to attack.

But unlike the Magpies who gave up after nesting the other tormentors were there all year round. The tormentors all ways found a new way to torment me but I never respond in kind. To retaliate. But I never showed them they were getting to me. I would go so far as to thank my tormentors because of their callous treatment I became a stronger person. I would not have been able to cope with the pain which I have had to suffer through my life. They may have thought they were having fun at my expense but I became tough and strong willed. Able to cope with what life had to dished out to me. Other wise I may have turned into a weak willed cry baby who didn't know how to handle loss, sickness, death, mental and physical abuse and come out on top.

One afternoon when I walked home I hung back because I knew my tormentors were planning to play a joke on me. On reaching a gum tree near an old tumble down building which had at one stage been a butcher shop, the group of them stopped to urge two of the group who were aboriginal boys, to show me something to try to make me sick. There was no way past them unless I took for the bush to get around them, that would be showing them I was chicken. Or scared of what they might do to me. In the future the pranks would have gotten worse. I kept walking and about to pass them by with out showing any interest in what they were doing.

Ruth Macklin

"Have you seen anyone eat witchetty grubs?" someone asked, trying to get my attention.

I had every intention of walking by with out taking any notice of them until a couple stepped in front of me to block my passage.

"Show her how you eat them,another edged the boys on. Most of my tormentors were older than the rest so should have had more sense than to be part of the game to get at me.

The witchetty grub was pulled from the tree, placed in the boy? mouth and swallowed. All I could imagine in my mind was the fine hairs tickling his throat as the live animal passed down to the stomach. Feel the grub crawling around inside his stomach. The thought made my stomach churn but I kept it down. No way was I going to be sick in front of them to show how weak I was. I shrugged my shoulders. Gave them all a disgusted look and turned to walk away from them. All the way home I wanted to be sick but I focused my mind on something else until the feeling had gone away. Not that I ate much dinner that night.

Ruth Macklin

Chapter Five

Then further into my school years my tormentors played other games, which they though would break my spirit but it didn't happen. One would be sent to befriend me so she could go back to her friends to tell them what had been said. I knew what their game was so I just went along with them to find what was next on their list. When the younger children started school I played with them to help them ease into being at school. They were not corrupted by the older students of the school. I watched Them play with their cars in the sand pit. Made sure they didn't lose them. This new peaceful life for me did not last long.

The first I knew of the trouble I was going to be in happened when we went back into class after out big lunch break. I knew I had not done anything wrong. My conscience was clear. But I was the fall guy. I was blamed and accused of theft.

"Sir! One of my toy cars is missing. I can't find it," said one of the young boys.

"Where did you see it last?"

"We were playing in the sandpit. It's not there now."

"Did you have a good look for it?" The boy nodded he did.

"Who was playing with you?"

"I was playing with him," .he pointed to the boy who had been playing cars with him.

"Any one else?"

"Yes. She was there with us," he finger was pointed at me.

"Did you take his car?" the teacher asked trying to get to the bottom of the stolen car so we could begin class.

"No, Sir." I knew I was innocent.

One hand went up. The person was asked what they wanted. The finger was pointed at me once again. "I saw Ruth put it in her school bag."

I was stunned! I couldn't believe they could stoop so low.

"Go out and bring you bag in side," I was ordered by the teacher.

I knew it would not be in there. I hadn't put anything my bag. I put the bag on the teacher's table and had to empty the contents on to the table. There, right at the bottom of my bag was the missing car. The one's who had placed the car in my bag their faces shone with glee. They had finally got the best of me they thought.

As I placed all my things back in my bag I straightened my spine to harden myself against what I knew would be my punishment. I was lucky in some ways because I was a girl. Boys were given the cane. Or cuts as they were called. Either across the open palm of their hand or they had to bend over to get the cane across their backside. I knew some boys who used to wear hair oil in their hair so they could put it on their hand to make the cane slip off with out hurting too much. That is, until the teacher woke up to what was

Ruth Macklin

happening.

The disgrace of being called a thief was worse to me than getting the cane. Especially when I did not commit the crime. I was made to write out line which said "I must not steal" a hundred times. But I took my punishment with out trying to clear my name because it would have been my word against all the others in the school. My tormentors did not hear a complaint from me. Nor did I shed a tear. All the trouble they went to they still did not break my spirit. It made my spirit stronger. It hardened me to face a lot of trouble fate had to send in my direction. I became steel on the inside to fight back in my own way, and time.

Another problem we had when we lived in the caravan was from a dog ,which belonged to my Aunt and Uncle. They lived in a house on the hill near the corrugated iron church. The shortest way to the house was along the railway line and over a wooden bridge. The road snaked around under the railway bridge and up the hill. The family had this big dog called Rover. Rover didn't like staying at his home. He wanted to come up to where our caravan was to sleep on the ground beneath the caravan in the cool. There was a big problem with him doing that. Rover had fleas. The fleas loved the cool, moist soil beneath the caravan. The fleas multiplied before the fleas invaded the caravan. No matter how many times we chased Rover out from under the caravan to send him home he always returned. Maybe it was quieter at our place.

Then one day my father got mad about the fleas. The toy I had made out of a Milo tin

Ruth Macklin

became the answer to the big small problem. The Milo tin had a nail hole in the lid and

the bottom. A length of wire had been threaded through the holes. Before the lid could be

hammered on the tin had to be filled with a lot of small stones, not over packed as the

stones had to have room to move. Rattle. The wire was connected together then a length

of string tired to the wire. When the tin was pulled along the ground the stones inside

rattled to make a lot of noise. It may not have been an expensive toy but it was something

to play with when you didn't have much else.

My toy just happened to be handy when my father got mad at Rover. Rover was called

and encouraged to come out from beneath the caravan. He was caught. The string of the

tin was tied to the tail of Rover. He was shooed to make him head for home. As Rover

ran the stones in the tin made a noise. Rover didn't take the long way home by the way of

the road which would have been better for him. He took the short cut along the railway

line. The noise from the stones inside the tin plus the tin bouncing on the blue metal over

the sleepers and the train rails, made Rover run all the faster. As Rover raced across the

walk way over the bridge the noise echoed. It would have sounded as though the Hounds

of Hell were hot on his heels. Rover was really travelling by the time he reached his

home. He flew in under the high blocked house to hide in the bath room. My Aunt had to

do a quick step to get out of the road or get knocked over by the dog. She was not very

happy with what had been done to Rover but he never again strayed from home. He was

cured of his wonder lust. I had to wait for another empty Milo. Or milk tin, to make

Ruth Macklin

another toy to play with.

After some time my uncle got a transfer to Bundaberg and my father applied for the job which was now vacant, got it, then we moved into the house on the hill. It was strange living in a house after years of living in tents, sheds and caravans. There was so much room it seemed like it was a castle. I finally had a room of my own. A large bed. It may have been bought second hand but the bed was a double size. I had heaps of room to roll around. Not the table size bed I had in the caravan. I didn't have to get out of my bed any more so we could make the bed into a table to eat on.

The house had four bedrooms, a closed in verandah and a kitchen with a wood stove. There was a problem with owning a wood stove because it made all the walls and ceilings smoked. My uncle got sick of trying to keep the ceiling clean so he decided to paint the ceiling a colour which would not show the smoke. He did not care if the new colour suited the rest of the kitchen. No one would ever see the smoked ceiling ever again. He would not have to keep cleaning it. Have a guess? You may have got it right. He painted the ceiling a lovely dark shade of black. The glow from the handy light no longer reflected from the white ceiling. The black had made the kitchen look darker.

Moving was a big job. All our belonging had to be taken out of the caravan to the house. Furniture had to be bought. The day we moved the furniture was fun but hard work. The men from the gang helped to carry the heavy stuff up the high steps into the house. Most of them helped except for one man. Another one of my uncles who had just

Ruth Macklin

returned back to camp from Bundaberg by the train. During the weekend he had been

drinking. Rum was his favourite drink. The drink was still in his system. Not that he

showed any signs of being hung over. He had helped carry some of the heavy items up the

steps. The last item he helped with was the fridge.

While my father knelt on the floor to light the wick of the fridge to get it cold to put in

the food, my uncle lent against the wall near the fridge and was soon fast asleep. He stood

there snoring. His legs didn't give away. The rest of the men carried on doing the work

and left him standing there out of the way until all the heavy pieces were in the house.

Someone tapped my uncle on the shoulder to wake him when the work was finished.

"What are you doing sleeping? We need a hand to get the work finished."

"I was not sleeping," came an indignant reply.

"Of cause you were. You were snoring. We all heard you."

"I was not sleeping. I was just resting my eyes." Everyone shook their head in

disbelief. They couldn't believe he had stood there so long sleeping without buckling at

the knees to slide down the wall to the floor.

We had to bath in the room under the house. The floor was cement but the walls were

still made from corrugated iron fixed to the posts with a wooden door. The water was still

cold. It came from the rainwater tanks at the side of the house. If you wanted to have a

warm bath you either had to light the copper, or boil water in a tin, or kettle, on the stove

and carry it down the steps to pour into the bath tub. A real bath tub. On hot days you

Ruth Macklin

could put some water in the tub and lay back to soak. The only draw back came at night

when you carried the handy light down the steps to go to the bathroom. The dreaded Cane

Toads would be waiting under the house to chase you as you carried the light to get to the

insects.

One night my mother and I were going down to have a bath after my father had

finished. My mother went first with the handy light and her clothes and I was not far

behind when the Cane Toads began hopping towards us. I spun around and jumped over

the side of the steps near the bottom and scooted up a few more steps. My mother ran for

the bathroom with the light and stepped into the bath while my father was still bathing.

He wondered what all the yelling was about.

"What happened? Did you see a snake?"

"The cane toads are chasing us," my mother finally got out, still puffing from her run.

The light was still in her hand.

"Why didn't you just put the light on the ground and walk away? They only wanted the

insects. You could have slipped getting into the tub and we both could have been burnt."

"I just wanted to get away from those nasty things."

"Now they will all be in the bathroom."

"I shut the door so I don't think too many got in." My father got out of the bath tub,

dried himself, dressed and took the light out of the bathroom to find where the cane toads

were and chased them away with a broom. He stayed to watch to see none of them came

Ruth Macklin

back until we finished our bath and were on our way back up the steps.

After we had been there for some time my father applied to the railway to have the bathroom put up stairs in the spare room at the end of the kitchen. It was a lot warmer in the winter for having a bath because most of the house would be kept warm while the fire in the stove burned. We had a water tank put on the side of the stove so we had hot water for baths and washing dished. We had to watch the tank was kept full of water so it wouldn't boil dry.

The toilet also was up graded to a wooden structure which stood on posts to keep out the water when it rained. And the Cane Toads as long as you did not forget to closed the door on your way out but the frogs were another problem. You could not keep them out. They would crawl up the wall and come over the space between the wall and the roof. You just had to search before you went in side and shut the door. The trip to the toilet, or out house, was cold in the winter and wet when it rained.

I am very pleased we now have inside toilets. Most of the places we had to live either had no toilet and you had to head for the bushed to find a safe, secure place, where there were no nasties, or people to watch what you were doing. But the worst one I ever had to use was the one my grandmother had at her house. A well type hole would be dug in the ground. The wooden out house would be placed over the top of the hole. When you lifted the lid to look for nasty surprised under the seat all you could see was this big, dark hole, feet deep. Once the hole was close to the top another hole was dug and the building

Ruth Macklin

moved to be placed over the new hole. I was very pleased when she finally moved and I did not have to go to that black hole of a toilet.

After we had been there in the house for awhile my father bought an engine to make 32volt electricity to run lights in the house instead of having to carry around handy lights where ever we went. The engine run each might to keep the batteries charged to run the lights when the engine had been turned off. We could even run a television on the batteries once television reached the country. The only draw back was I had to learn to crank the engine to get it started when my father was not at home. You had to let the handle go quick once it kicked and started. You also had to let go quick when the engine kicked back. If you didn't you were looking at a broken arm, or something more serious. The trip to the doctor would have been slow, and very painful.

The lighting plant consisted of an engine with a big wheel. A wide flat belt went from the big wheel to a generator which charged all the batteries connected together on the bench. Each battery was connected together with alligator clips on the end of a short piece of wire. On the side of the big wheel there was a handle which you pulled out to use to wind the wheel around to get the engine to kick to start it. I had to concentrate the engine gave the right kick not the one where I had to get my hand out of the way quickly.

On the wall was another way to start the engine as long as I had not let the batteries go to long without charging them. I think it was a type of points system where I had to use a short stick to reach across the bench to reach a special gadget on this piece of wood. I'll

Ruth Macklin

push on the gadget which would make the wheel turn to start the engine. I had to be a quick learner or would have to go with out lights when at home on my own. The engine had to be filled with fuel and the oil checked out before the engine could be started. I had to watch the points didn't stick when the engine started other wise I would have to stop the engine and try once again.

Berajondo was a good place for character building. You grew tough. Or you sank to the very bottom of despair. Most of the time I had to find things to keep myself occupied by doing different kinds of jobs, riding my bicycle, or laying on my stomach beside a water hole, or drain, dangling a length of cotton, or string into the water with a piece of meat on the end. I learned patience by this time consuming game. How to be quiet. To pull up the line with a slow, steady hand and be slow and quick to get the container beneath the line to catch the lobbies before they let go of the meat and disappeared back to their holes in the mud. Doing this filled in a lot of hours once it had rained and the lobbies came up from being buried deep in the ground. Once the water finally dried up I had to find another hole or wait until it rained once again. Some places where the water was shallow I could walk through the water lifting up stones to see if there were any lobbies hiding beneath them.

We could also go fishing down in Baffle creek. The only problem with that idea we had to take a shovel, or maddock with to dig for worms to put on the hooks to catch the fish. We would drive to the bank of the creek and find a sandy area on which to stand to

Ruth Macklin

fish when the tide was out but had to move quick once it began to come in again. Then we would have to sit on the grassy bank where there were a lot of trees. The trees were a big problem. Twirling the line to throw it out into the water the hook would catch on the branches of the trees then we would have to pull hard in the hope the branch broke. Or the line broke.

Sitting beside the river was so peaceful and quiet. So relaxing. The sound of the water lapping against the bank. The birds singing in the trees. We were shaded from the hot sun by the tall trees. I could sit there for hours waiting for the fish to bite the bait. The thrill of pulling hard on the line to drag the fish to the bank before it let go. Or it headed to where there was a snag in the water and you would have to break the line to get it free. Once it was snagged we would hold the line tight and turn our body slowly to strain the line until it let go, or snapped. We had to watch we didn't fall over once it gave way. Or got stung with the line when it snapped.

There were only three kinds of fish I didn't like to catch. The Catfish which stung with its spikes which were very painful. Eels were another. We had to keep them away from the line on the ground once they had been landed because they would slither all over the ground and tangle up the line. The line would take ages to get it untangled. Nearly as bad as getting the line in a bunch of grapes. A bunch of grapes was when the line got all tangled and we had to have patience to sit there to untangle it. If you didn't have the patience the bunch of grapes were cut off and new tackle put at the end of the cut. We

Ruth Macklin

took the knotted piece of line home where we sat at leisure to patiently untangle the line to use another day. The third fish was of the Stone Fish variety but lives in fresh water and is called a bullrout which has three sacks of venom on its spines. That is not what my father called it. Many a times he called it a lot of unmentionable names especially when he had been stung by the wrong fin. We would have to drive for Bundaberg to get a couple of needles for the pain.

Ruth Macklin

Chapter Six

Over the other side of Baffle Creek and up on the slight rise there was a fresh water

lagoon. A lagoon where most things, which went into the water didn't come out, so the

stories go. This place where we used to go to pump water into forty-four gallon drums to

take back to the caravan, and later the house, when the rain water tanks were low. The

lagoon was a very quiet place surrounded with trees except for the side near the road. The

ground was of clay type soil where only a few trees grew. All the years I live there the

lagoon never went dry. The level of the water dropped a bit but never went dry. There

were a few reeds near the side where we parked the truck to pump the water. Perch lived

in the water. No birds, to my knowledge, ever swam on the surface of the water. They

would perch on the dead tree in the water but that was all they did.

There was something strange about the place. You felt like you were being watched

the whole time you were there. The ghostly feelings which made you feel you had to

whisper when you spoke not to disturb what ever was watching. Cold shivers ran down

the spine. The imagination of a ten year old worked over time. Even when I reached

fourteen I could still feel the presence of unseen life in the water. Or you could say the

Bunyip had a close eye on all who dared to come to his home.

One day when my parents and I went to the lagoon to fill up the drums on the back of the truck I grabbed a short piece of garden hose off of the back of the truck. I lay down on

the ground near a tree to place the hose in the water to blow bubbles. It was a stupid place

for me to pick because the rain over time had been washing the clay soil away from

around the base of the tree. The water had also been eroding away the soil from under the

tree roots. As the hose had a slight bend I moved closed to the edge to get a better look at

the bubbles.

"Get away from there!my father shouted at me when he moved the hose from one

drum to the other. "Before you ...." was as far as he got before I toppled head first into the

water. The soil holding the roots system together fell away and the roots broke.

I should have known to keep away from the water. Never did like water where I could

not touch the bottom with my feet. My mother rushed to where I had fallen in to wait to

see if I surfaced. Or whether the Bunyip could have caught me. But at the time of my

falling into the lagoon I was not aware there were stories circulating around the district,

about the things which never came out of the lagoon. I was innocent of the fact I could

have been taken and not come back to the surface.

After a short time I reached the surface spluttering to get the water from my face. I

reached out blindly to grab a root of the tree. I was crying from the shock of falling into

the cool water even though the weather was warm. I rubbed one hand over my face to get

rid of the water. Weed and green slime were in my hair. The slime slipping down over my

face which made me cry all the more and want to get out of the water. I tried to kick my

legs as I pulled my way around the edge of the lagoon to where I knew the water would

Ruth Macklin

be shallow. I had a dip in the shallow bit once before. And only once because black, slimy leeches lived in the clay mud, which had clung to my legs. They were hard to get off.

I finally made it up on to the bank. Shaking my head to try to get rid of the slime, and weed, shivering with shock. My father had no sympathy for me. Told me it was my own stupid fault I had fallen in the lagoon. My mother tried to comfort me as she pulled the weed from my hair. I did not like the slime sliding down over my body.

"Move out of the way," my Mother was told. "I'll get her clean." As I had my back to the truck I did not know what my father had intended to do before I was nearly knocked off my feet by the blast of cold water from the hose, which he had been using to fill the drums. "Turn around." I turned to get the full force of the water on my head which I had bend forward to try to stop the water hitting me in the face. My dress clung to my body.

When the water had stopped hitting me I was going to get into the front of the truck because anyone could see through the material. I didn't want any one to see me wet. Not any of my tormentors if they happened to be driving past the lagoon.

"No you don't!" My father yelled as I went to climb up into the front of the truck. "You're not getting in there wet."

"I'll sit on the back with the drums," I replied, hoping the drums would hide me from prying eyes. But that was not to be either.

"You will be walking all the way home. It will teach you not to do things you shouldn't. You had better get started if you want to make it home before dark."

Ruth Macklin

I couldn't believe I had to walk home. It was a couple of miles. I would be ages getting

home. I thought my mother would stand up for me and make my father let me ride home

on the back of the truck. A dejected figure I sat on an old log in the sun in the hope my

clothes would be dry enough by the time the drums were all filled but that was not to be.

My parents got in the truck and drove away and left me sitting there. For a short time I sat

there hoping they would come back for me but the truck did not return. The sun began to

get lower in the sky. I had no intentions of spending the night in such a spooky place.

Standing up I looked in all directions to see if there were any cars coming along the

road. I walked to the edge of the road and listened for any sounds which might mean a

car, or truck, coming my way. Looked at the ground to see I did not step on any thing

which would make a noise to tell the spooks I was moving through their area, I crept

along the road which was another problem. All those trees which came right up close to

the edge of the road. So close together you could not see if there were any people, or

animal, waiting to grab a young girl as she tried to pass. There was no place for me to run

to if a car came along.

Slowly I made my way down the hill keeping a close eye on the trees. Then there was

the bridge to cross. The long, rattly, wooden planked bridge with no where to go if a car,

or truck, came charging down the hill and around the corner to cross the bridge. If I stood

on the wrong plank it would rattle and echo up and down the river. Surveying the bridge I

decided the best way to go was the planks which ran across the planks which went

Ruth Macklin

sideways. They looked as though they would not make so much noise. I listened for

noise. There was none. It was now, or never. There was only one way to go. I lined up

with one of the planks. Double checked for traffic. Then I ran as fast as I could to get to

the other side of the bridge and past the trees on the other side before any traffic could

come. With the feeling of being watched as I ran I pushed myself to run faster not even

feeling the stone hurting my bare feet until I had reached safety on the other side. A stitch

of pain grabbed me in my right side as I topped the hill on the other side and I kept going

until I could go no further. I made it to the side of the road and collapsed on the bank of

the drain taking deep breaths to try to get the pain to go away. When I finally felt a little

better I began to walk the rest of the way home.

As I walked home I listened for cars and kept changing to the other side of the road

when there was the more shelter on that side, such as trees, mounds of dirt, gullies and

long grass, so I could hide from who ever came along. I didn't want a story about me

spread around. "Stupid Ruth had fallen in the lagoon," my tormentors would laugh and

make fun of me. A couple of times I had to dive for cover. By the time I had reached the

old hotel I was nearly dry. I sat on the back steps for awhile which were not used much

any more. I walked up behind the hotel passed behind the hall to cut through a paddock,

then I quickly climbed through the fence out on to the road at the top of the hill, across

the road to go through the railway paddock where sleepers and other timbers were stored

waiting to be loaded on to wagons to be railed away. From there I had to walk down the

wooden steps fashioned into the side of the bank for people to get to the railway station to be able to collect their mail. I crossed the railway line and finally made it home with out

being caught wet.

Because we all liked seafood, when my father was not working he like to travel to the

coast where he could catch crabs, fish and prawns. The best part was in the eating. The

worst parts were we had to get up in the dark to travel hours over rough, non-existent

roads to get to the best place to get the crabs. The roads were mostly goat tracks through

peoples properties to get to these places. These days there has been roads built for the

tourists to get to the area where we had to slog through the bush to get there. Drive over

wet, muddy flats when it had been raining. Some areas were swamp. Either very high

tides crossed the road or rain made it hard to cross. We had to walk the road in places to

find where the road was hard and try to drive the car over the hard ground without

slipping into the soft ground. If the car spun into the soft ground we had to get out to

either push the car, or dig our way out.

One day that is what we had to do. The car spun and down went the four wheels into

he soft mud. The chassis of the car sat on the hard section of the road. When the engine

was revved the wheels spun mud and water flying in all directions. We all had to get out

of the car. Luckily my father had come prepared. A shovel and axe were unloaded. My

father and his friend took turns at digging as much mud away from in front, and behind

the wheels, to place pieces of old trees beneath the wheels. The wood was packed in the

slush for the wheels to get traction to get the car to move. When it was packed some of

Ruth Macklin

the mud was pushed away from the middle to let the wheels sit on the packing.

My father got into the car while the rest of us gave a hand to push the car to get it moving. As the wheels spun to get traction the mud came flying back to cover us from head to toe. We were all ready half muddy but by the time the car was out we were completely covered. We 'd slip and slide through the mud to get to the car. Before getting in the car we would try to remove as much of the mud as we could, except for our clothes, then continue on to the beach where we could clean up. My father and his friend did not clean up until it was time to go home as they spent most of the day trailing around in the mud until they had caught enough crabs to take home. Or until the incoming tide chased them back to the beach.

My mother and I would make our way to the edge of the water to sit down to wash away some of the mud before to dried too much and caked on to the skin, and clothes, which was a silly idea really. We should have kept covered with the mud so the sand flies did not bite us so much. While we waited near the car we would go trailing through the mud flat looking for crabs. At certain times of the year the crabs beached themselves and we would nearly stand on them not knowing they were covered with the mud. We learnt to carry a stick to search the mud so we did not step on them. I would hold them down with the stick and my mother would tie a string around them so we would not get bitten if the crabs stuck the points of their claws through the mesh of the bag.

Playing with crabs is very dangerous. Once they have clamped their claw on to

Ruth Macklin

something they will not let go, even when they throw their claw. The claw still hangs

tight. My father was not quite quick enough one day. The crabs lifted its claws and got his

finger. He cursed and swore with the pain. We tried to get the crab to let go but it

wouldn't. We all thought the finger would be missing when it finally let go. It is safe to

say the finger was still in tact. But there were not many recognisable parts of the crab left

as it was smashed against the nearest tree. The claw still clamped to his finger. A stone

had to be found to smash the claw to get the finger out. The three of us were expecting to

have to make a mad, slow, long dash to the nearest hospital with a finger missing. The

finger survived to work another day. The skin was not even broken but the finger was

badly bruised and sore for days. Just as well because someone had to get us back through

the boggy place.

Lucky for us on both accounts my father still had his finger. He couldn't afford to lose

any more. And the sun had been shining brightly, and hot, so the ground had dried out

some where we had been bogged. The slush had dried out and held the logs together for

us to get through. The sun had gone down by the time we had arrived back home. Once

the car had been unpacked my father set about placing wood beneath the copper to light a

fire while his mate filled the copper with water in which to cook the crabs. While we

waited for the water to come to the boil, we took turns in the bath getting cleaned up. To

wash away the salt water and the remnants of the mud from our hair, and body.

Once the water began to bubble merrily, the crabs were placed into the water and salt

added, then while they cooked we had something to eat. The smell of the crabs took away

Ruth Macklin

our liking for too much other food. We only ate enough to hold us over until the first

batch of crabs could be lifted from the boiling water. A shovel was used to lift the crabs

out of the water then they were placed on to a piece of corrugated iron to cool. The next

batch would be put in. We sat around the copper watching, and waiting, for the crabs to

be cool enough to start to eat them while they were still warm. I suppose that way of

eating crabs spoilt me for not wanting to eat a crab which has not just been taken from the

boiling water. They have a better taste than those which have been cooked and allowed to

cool.

The same with prawns, I love the prawns which have been cooked and can be eaten as

soon as they are cool enough to handle. After chasing around trying to catch them as the

net is dragged up on to the beach and getting dug by their spikes, you seem to get more

enjoyment out of the eating than if you went to the shop to buy them. Even the sunburn

and the sand flies are forgotten while you enjoy the fruits of the chase to catch as many as

you can before they return back to the water.

Another place where we went fishing we had to go across a rocky area which looked

like the surface of the moon, or melon holes in the rocks. Maybe the melon holes

happened from years of the tidal water passing over the rocks. Or there was another

reason. The car rocked, and bumped, through the dips in the rocks to get to the other side.

On the top side of the rocks the water was deep and a good place to catch Cod Fish so we

had been told.

Ruth Macklin

The car was parked on the other side. We got out our lines and bait. In those days the lines were on reels. They were fine when fishing from a sandy place but not too good while fishing from a grassy bank. The line would tangle in the weeds and grass. On this occasion, my line got tangled in the weeds once I had pulled it in to re-bait the hook. I was tired. We had been to what was called a kitchen tea for a friend who would soon to be married. It was midnight by the time we had arrived home from the dance hall. My father dragged us back out of bed before the sun had gotten out of bed. I opened bleary eyes to try to look at the time on my watch I had forgotten to take of when we arrived home but it was too dark to see the time.

Things seemed to happen quick. I had thrown out the line. Forgotten to place my foot on the reel on the ground. When the baited hook hit the water so did my reel. I got down on my knees near the edge to reach out to get the reel before it had a chance to float away. Next minute I was in the water. I suddenly came fully awake as I went under the water. I had to be dragged out this time because there was no way I could have climbed out on my own. The worse part of the falling in I still had on my new watch I had been given for Christmas. It never went again. By the afternoon the salt water had started to eat, and rust, all the mechanical parts of the watch. There was not a piece of it which was capable of ever working again. I don't know why I seem to keep falling into deep water. Maybe it was a sign to warn me of all the trouble which I had to face as I travelled through life.

Ruth Macklin

It was good living in the house on the hill. I had a swing under the house this time because there were no trees suitable to hang the rope from. The rope was tied to the timber which went across the top of the posts. Strips of tarpaulin were nailed to the posts to try to keep some of the rain out of the things which were kept under the house. The car, tools and the bench where my father worked when fixing engines, or chainsaw.

One area between two posts I stacked the fire wood so I would not have to travel down to the wood heap in the dark to fetch more wood for the fire, or copper. Most of the stack stayed dry when it rained. Only the bottom couple of layers got wet as the rain water flowed through under the house. The stack was always kept full. When my father went in search of fire wood, he made sure he found the softest of timber. He had plenty of years practice with cutting timber. Now he was cutting fire wood to take to people who owned wood stoves. Even trucked it all the way to Bundaberg. This was how my parents filled in the weekends when we were not going fishing. The farmers got their paddocks cleared of old fallen timber this way.

I stayed home while they went cutting fire wood so there would be a cooked meal waiting when they arrived home. To fill in some of my time during the day I would go down to the wood heap and split the blocks up into pieces which would fit into the fire box. Most times it took one strike with the axe and the piece would go flying off the block. I would keep turning the block to a different position then took another swipe until the block was all in pieces. As I worked the pieces of wood were thrown on to a pile.

Ruth Macklin

When I thought I had chopped enough for the day I would load up the wheelbarrow with wood to wheel up to the house to stack it. It was so peaceful working along at my own pace. My father did not have to cut much wood for the fire unless there were some hard blocks. It was one less job he had to do. Except he had to keep changing the handle in the axe. The way I chopped the handle seemed to come off the worst. Hitting the wood with the handle when the block slipped ate away the handle until it broke.

Ruth Macklin

Chapter Seven

To my way of think of what I had to do over the years, I had become my Father's son as well as my Mother's daughter. I was his T.A. (Another way of saying I was his helper in the messy jobs.) Like when the engine in the cars broke. From the time I could find, or hold a spanner, I had to help. Given the hard, time consuming work once the engine was out on the ground and pulled to pieces. The pistons were the hardest. The caked on carbon on the top of the piston had to be chipped away with a chisel, or screwdriver and scrubbed with a steel brush once the part had spent a bit of time soaking in petrol. The grooves around the side of the piston where the rings were placed to keep the piston tight in the bore had to have the dirt gouged out so the new rings fitted snug. Very time consuming and boring.

When I was not cleaning I had to find spanners or hold the lead light, or torch, for my father to see what he was doing as we worked well into the night to get the car fixed. A ramp had been built down near the wood heap. There was space under the ramp for my father to work beneath the car without having to use any jacks. A block and tackle hung from a branch of the tree to help raise the engine out of the car once the bonnet had been removed. It seemed to me every time one of our cars, or one of the engines used for cutting timber had broken, I was the only one available to do all the dirty, hateful jobs.

Ruth Macklin

Everyone else needed to be somewhere else. My father, and I, work on cars for friends but they were no where to be found until the work on our car had been completed. But they were the first ones there to get a ride in the car if they wanted to go the same way we were going. A fair amount of my life was being my father's T.A. When I was available. Once I left home my mother had to help where she could.

The parts if they were not spotless and shining, I had to go back to the scrubbing until there were no bits of dirt on the parts. Even a tiny bit of dirt and the pieces would not fit back together properly. Many a day while engines were being fixed I worked well into the night to have the parts ready to have the other pieces, like rings, added to them before they were tapped gently back into the bore. Other times I had to search for the spanners which went flying through the air because they would not do the job. Night time was the worse to look for greasy spanners in the dark.

Sometimes it was best to sleep on the problem and the next day everything would fit where it was suppose to, after a good night sleep. There would be no more cursing and shouting. There would be no blazing eyes shining at me from a face covered with splashes of oil and grease. I would just close my ears to the words which would turn the air blue at the time. I would just search for the missing things and keep helping where I could. Not that it was fun playing in grease and petrol. The hands would stink for days no matter how many times I washed them. The skin would become rough from all the hours spent in the petrol.

Ruth Macklin

Before the designs of the cars were changed I could tell what parts went into most engines. Or what could be wrong with the car. But now it is not safe to look under the bonnet because there are not too many of the same parts. The body of the cars are made to fall to pieces with the slightest of bumps. They don't have a chassis to hold them together when the car is involved in an accident. The driver seems to get all the blame, or road conditions. Cars, like most other products, are not made to last. Things are made to fall apart so we have to keep spending our money to replace them so keeping the worker poor and in debt.

Going off to high school was another experience. The year was the first year grade eight became a high school grade in Queensland. Our class room consisted of four walls put around the stumps beneath the state school. The school stood on high blocks which had cement on the ground where the primary students kept their bags, and where we played if the weather was wet. Part of the walls were glass. There were about twenty of us in the class room under the school. We came from all different parts of the surrounding country side. We were driven to school in an old Holden station wagon. Just as well there were no seat belt rules in those days because we were packed into the car like sardines, children and bags.

In the car which started from Lowmead there were eight students plus the driver. Three more of us got in at Berajondo. How the owner of the car ever got away with having so many of us in the car I don't know? For the whole of the school year we

Ruth Macklin

travelled in that car. How we were not killed was a miracle. If the car had ever been run through a road worthy it would never have passed. But no one complained about the way their children had to travel miles to school in an unsafe car. Some had to travel ten miles or more to and from school. Luckily I was only in the car for five of those miles. The last ones in, and the first ones out, got to have the seats with some of the others. The rest had to squeeze into the baggage compartment at the back. Come to think of it, I don't remember even seeing a tool box in case the car broke down. There were no mobiles to call for help if help was needed. We would have had to sit there and wait for a car to come along to get some help for us.

The car was always on the move so I don't know how it ever got serviced. How it held together for so long without breaking down. On one occasion when it rained we had to leave school before the creeks came up. Us Berajondo three got home early but the rest of the students had to take the long way home. They had to go around the back roads which added hours on to the trip to get to Lowmead. The fluid in the brakes ran low so the driver replaced the brake fluid with muddy, rain water, to have brakes to be able to keep driving the car to get home. Not that the water in the brake line would have done good to the workings of the car. After I heard of what had happened I was always thankful when I made it home alive, and in one piece. We just held on and prayed we would get to where were were meant to be. Maybe the ones who talked a lot, or joked around, only done that because they were scared of not making their destination.

Ruth Macklin

Going to Rosedale school was a better proposition. There were more students from

different towns and they were not all related. Or long time family friends so they mixed

with everyone. The year there was more peaceful. More friendly. I at least had some

students which I could call my friends. Some of the younger classes liked to tease us

because we had to have the class room under the school but it was done in fun. I started to

enjoy going to school.

I would have liked to go on to further my education but I was not allowed by my

parents. Also I had my tonsils taken out a couple of days after New Year's Day. There

was no problem getting them out. The operation went well. I was given the old type

aesthetic where a mask thing was placed over the nose and drops of Chlorophyll dropped

on the mask. I had a feeling of being suffocated. Not being able to breathe. I wanted to

fight to get the mask off my nose. My face was going numb. I wanted to lift my arms to

try to get rid of the thing causing me so much distress but my arms did want to work with

the brain. That was the last I remember until I woke up back in my bed.

My parents were worried about me having the operation. They had tried for years to

have a doctor to take out my tonsils but the doctors would not do the operation. ?our

daughter is a bleeder. She may bleed to death during the operation. ?hey had never tested

me to see if that was the case. Maybe they were of the opinion people with reddish hair

were all bleeders.

Then one night when I was very sick with my tonsils, my mother had driven us to

Bundaberg to get me to the hospital but the car stopped near a doctor's surgery. The

doctor took me in and he explained to us why my very rotten tonsils had not been taken

out. The poison was spreading through out my body causing other problems. My teeth

had all ready had to be taken out at the top because they had decayed and broken.

"We'll have some tests done. This will tell us what we can do,The doctor gave me

tablets to get rid of the infection. My mother was told where to take me to have a blood

test done to confirm whether I was a bleeder, or not.

A couple of weeks later I had to go to have the blood test done. Blood was taken out of

my arm. I thought that was all I had to have done. Next a needle was dug into my ear lobe

and a piece of paper, like blotting paper, caught the drops of blood while the lady timed

the drops to see how long the blood took to stop. When the tests were in the doctor made

a time to have my tonsils out. He also gave me some tablets to make my blood thicker. In

the mean time my grandfather, my mother's father, died and was buried a couple of days

before I had to have the operation. My mother wanted to put off the operation but I

wanted to have it done so I would not have to miss so many days from school because of

illness.

The same day of the operation I was brought steak and eggs to have for dinner. I could

hardly talk let alone try to swallow steak no matter how soft it may have been. I went with

out. My parents came in to visit me not long after I came back to bed and my mother

nearly collapsed from the smell of the anaesthetic still on me. My father had to quickly

Ruth Macklin

get a chair for her to sit on before her legs buckled to let her fall to the floor.

After I returned home from the hospital I found I was not thinking clearly. Work which I had learnt at school the year before, and other things which happened before I went to the hospital, were gone. It seemed as though the aesthetic had cleaned some of the memory from my brain. I had hopes of my memory returning once I had returned to school but that was not to be. I didn't get the chance to go back to school. The option was not mine to make.

"When are we going shopping for my school books? asked my mother. It would take me days to get them all covered for school if I didn't get them very quickly.

"You won't be going back to school," I was told by my mother. "Girls don't need an education. They just get married and all that money spent on education is wasted. You will just have to find a job."

A job! How was I to get work? I lived about fifty miles from Bundaberg. There was no chance of me finding work in the country. I thought I may have a better chance if we lived closer to Bundaberg. I was not allowed to go to town to stay to find work. So I had to stay at home and continue to do work at home. Later in the year, my father put in for a transfer to Bundaberg which he go and we moved into town. I did get a few little jobs but I was not allowed to go too far away from home. I was offered a job of companion out west on a cattle station near Longreach but I was not allowed to go. Maybe if I had been allowed to travel out west for the job my life may have taken a different path. Maybe I would not

Ruth Macklin

have had to suffer so much.

I finally met a guy when I went out with a cousin. Like him a lot. Thought he was for me. But that was not to be. He told a few too many lies. Said he was going to go out of town so he would not be able to see me. I found out what he did instead. Him and his friends were with other girls. The next time I ran into him I told him just what I thought of him. Not very often I swore even though I had been around people who swore a lot. He thought he had not been found out and wanted to carry on as before. I walked away from him. Left him with his friends to console him. I ignored his attempts to talk to me. I should have learnt once burnt to keep away from guys.

But silly me found another guy. If I would have been thinking straight I should have run miles to get away from him. He was nothing but trouble from the beginning. He drank which I didn't. He smoked which I didn't. He had been in trouble with the law for stealing. The only part of my time with him which was any good was the birth of my two children. Along with him came the know-it-all mother-in-law. She knew everything. She was all ways right. Never wrong. Even when someone with more experience on the subject she was right and they were wrong.

She lived in a haunted house. I believed it was. Each time I walked into the house I could feel eyes watching me. Feel a presence close behind me. I didn't like to spend the night there. I came up with every excuse I could find not to sleep there. Like not enough beds. Don't like sleeping in strange houses. My excuses worked for a some time after we

Ruth Macklin

were married.

Not long after we were married our first child was born. A girl who we called her Jody. That was a mistake. I didn't spell the name right. It should have been Jodi. His mother was the one who said I had spelt it like a boy's name would be spelt. She was

mad because she had rushed out and bought a name brooch with the name spent Jodi. Her family consisted of only two sons she was now set on a course to spoil the granddaughter. She all ways jumped in to buy things. Especially if she knew my mother was intending to buy some little present, or clothes. It was a game of one up man's ship. In the end it felt as though I was in the middle of a tug-a-war. One complaining because the other kept sticking her nose in to try to get the situation to suit herself and no one else. I was the meat in the sandwich. If I said anything to my husband about what was happening I was harping.

"You just don't want my mother to have anything to do with Jody. She is her grandmother. She has as many rights as your mother. Your parents see Jody more than mine do. So I knew not to expect any help from my husband. I seemed to be the odd one out in the family. My opinion did not count for much. So I kept my own counsel. Did things my way when it came to looking after my daughter. I had looked after other people? children from about the age of nine so I knew what I was doing.

Jody could not use baby powder. It brought her out in a rash. I was told by the lady from the Health Clinic not to use the baby powder because it was what caused the rash.

Ruth Macklin

No. That was not the case. I didn't know what I was talking about.

"I used it on both my children and it never hurt them," raved his mother. "I've never heard of it causing a rash. It is made to use on babies. The company would not be able to sell it for babies if it harmed them. There's nothing wrong in using the baby powder."

She didn't think some babies, like adults, do have reactions to different products. Powder just happened to be one of the things she could not use all through her short life. But his mother still would not be told powder was the problem even when the rash went away from not using powder of any type.

At the time Jody was born we were living in a caravan in the railway yard where my husband was working. I had to boil all the clothes in a tin over a fire then rinse them out in a tub of water, wring them out by hand, then hang them on a piece of wire. It was hard, back breaking work for a person straight home from the hospital. Even before I went to the hospital it was hard enough doing our clothes the same way. I had to do all the work. The pub was just a short walk across the paddock. I was not very happy I was again living in a caravan trying to raise a baby.

We moved from place to place as he was transferred. On one of our returns to Bundaberg I became very sick with some type of cold. We were staying at my parent? house but they were away on holiday. With each day which passed I got worse and could not look after anyone. He complained it was too much to look after the both of us. My husband and his mother ganged up on me. Next I knew it had all been arranged. I was

Ruth Macklin

bundled into the car and taken to the haunted house to sleep. We were given the double

bed in the master bedroom. Even though as sick as I was I did not want to be there in that

house. Didn't want to have to sleep in their room. But I was not given any say in the

matter. I know I was very ill. I thought I was going to die. Staying in that house was a

living nightmare.

I believe I would have gotten better quicker if I had stayed where I was. The

nightmares were a living hell. I didn't want to be there. The Avenger of Darkness was

there in the room. He was there every time I closed my eyes. I twisted and turned in bed

trying to get away from him. I pleaded to be taken away from that house. Didn't want to

die there. She was there in the wings waiting for me to die to take my baby away from me

to keep for her own. Her thinking was she could do a better job of raising my daughter

than I could.

Each time I closed my eyes, which was often once the doctor was called. I kept

floating around the house in my sleep keeping an eye on Jody. Had to make sure she was

still in the house and not taken away while I was ill. I never slept soundly. Each morning I

was exhausted from keeping watch over my daughter. While I was floating around in the

air like a bird the Avenger of Darkness was there chasing me. I could fly like a bird. My

arms were used for wings. My arms were all ways tired and sore each morning as I

returned to my body on the bed. My whole body would be exhausted. All through the

night I had been chased through the air where I tumbled, turned, soared and hid, to get

Ruth Macklin

away from the Avenger of Darkness.

For well over a week I could not sleep properly. Every night I left my body behind in the bed to travel through the air keeping watch over my daughter. Watched over my own body to make sure no one removed it while I was not there. I was afraid my body would be missing and I would not be able to return to it when the morning came for me to return. I didn't trust anyone in the house. If they only knew I was missing at night my body would have been taken away. If my body was not there to return to I knew I would be left floating forever haunting the house, being chased by the Avenger of Darkness for ever. I would be dead. But I couldn't die. I was too young to die. I was only nineteen years of age. The mother-in-law would have been pleased because she would have fought tooth and nail to get custody to have Jody as her own.

With the thought of her taking care of my daughter I fought hard to return to health. To recover from what type of bug had taken over my body. I was not going to die just to please her. I had a mission in life now. Even though I had this feeling when I was growing up that I would only live to the age of twenty. Thankfully I am still here today. As I keep saying now I am lucky to have lived past my idea of used by date. I will keep fighting until I don't have the energy to fight. Until my mission here on Earth has been completed.

As soon as I was able to get out of bed and able to walk around enough I was out of the house and back over to my parent's house. A place where I could have a good night's

Ruth Macklin

sleep without being chased all night. A restful sleep which would help my body heal quickly. A place I didn't have to worry about the Avenger of Darkness and the ghosts who followed me all the time I was in that house. No way would I have recovered so quickly if I had not moved out of the haunted house.

Ruth Macklin

Chapter Eight

Once we had moved hundred of miles away from Bundaberg, I thought our lives would be better. There would be no more interference. No more family hassles. None of his drinking buddies would be around. We would live in peace. We would have more money. We wouldn't have to worry where we were going to get money from ti live, and pay our bills. That was a joke. Even with the higher wages the money seemed to disappear.

We lived in the caravan in one of the caravan parks in Townsville. A small bed for Jody had been built into the caravan. It was not an ideal place because we had to keep the window locked all the time so she would not play with the catches to get out the window. She didn't seem to happy with the bed even though she was only one year old. She showed us in a not very nice way her dislike of the bed. Even at such a young age she was very strong willed when she wanted her own way.

One day Jody was asleep so I went over to the toilet but when I returned I knew she had woken because she had her face to the window as I walked into the annex. There was something on her face. I rushed in to see what she had gotten into. The smell hit me as I opened the caravan door. She had dirtied her nappy and it had fallen out. The wall and curtains near her bed had been plastered with poo. It was on her face and hands from where she had been playing in it. The smell, and the sight of the mess churn my stomach

Ruth Macklin

but I held it down with great difficulty.

The first job was to get Jody clean before she could do any more painting of the walls. She seemed so happy with the job she had done. Not too happy when she had to have a bath and hair wash to get rid of the poo off her. She cried and fought to get out of the bathtub. When she had been cleaned and dressed I placed her on the double bed where I could keep an eye on her while I worked. The curtains had to be removed to be washed. All her sheets and pillow slip had to be washed. They were taken out into the annex to soak in buckets of water. I then had the task of washing the walls to remove the art work and the smell. It took ages to get it off because it had dried while I had been cleaning her, and feeding her in between the jobs.

One of her other turns had us frightened. I didn't think what I was doing but what I did worked. I believe it saved her life. Jody had finished eating her meal. I cleaned her up. Took her from her high chair and placed her in her bed while we washed the dishes from our meal. She did not want to be put in bed. She was only put there until we could do the cleaning up and she would not be in the way. We just thought she had stopped crying and was playing. Jody was too quiet. The shock I go when I turned from putting dishes in the cupboard had me racing to her.

Jody had gone blue. In her temper she had held her breath. She was not breathing. When I lifted her from the bed she went limp in my arms. I had remembered some stories about wetting their face to bring them around. I tried talking to her. Then I remembered

Ruth Macklin

another thing to do. I laid her on the bed and grabbed her by the feet. I lifted her up by the

ankles and gently lowered her upside down. I lowered her and raised her gently a few

time until the up and down motion made her gasp and start to breath. Once she had taken

her first breath I laid her down on the bed then picked her up to cuddle her until she

stopped crying. She finally cried herself to sleep. At intervals during the night I kept

getting up to watch she was sleeping peacefully and not sick from holding her breath. I

kept a close eye on her from then on to make sure she did not try the same thing again.

Jody didn't do it for me but she tried the same thing on my mother who was bathing her.

She didn't want to get out of the bath so began to hold her breath. She got a face washer

full of water in the face which brought her out before she could pass out again.

Not long after that episode I started getting sick once again. Didn't take much notice at

first. Just thought it was the gastric and vomiting which had been going through the

caravan park. I could not eat because nothing would stay down, not even a drink of water.

Once my stomach was empty I didn't have to make so many trips across the park to the

toilet but I had to lay on the bed with my head over a bucket. My husband was working so

I had to look after Jody as well. I finally took my self to the hospital to get some

medicine. I finally go in to see the doctor who took blood tests and gave me some

medication. I don't know how but I got Jody back to the car and drove home where I went

back to bed but as the day wore on I had gotten worse. Had to have Jody on the bed with

me because I could not lift her. Had to drag myself around the caravan by holding on to

the cupboards to get food for her. By the late afternoon I was completely exhausted with

Ruth Macklin

no energy at all.

"I want you to take me back to the hospital,? mumbled when my husband walked through the door of the caravan.

"I thought you were going this morning. Didn't you go?"

"I did. But I want you to take me back. Put some clothes in a bag for me."

"Why? What did they say was wrong?"

"Just said I had a stomach bug. The doctor took some test and sent me home."

"They won't do anything more for you, now."

"Oh, yes they will. I'm taking clothes to stay in hospital. They won't be sending me home. I don't have the strength to move." My bag was packed and put into the car. Jody strapped in the car seat. I was then helped to make my way out of bed, through the caravan, nearly fell down the steps, and half walked and half dragged out to the car. Once I finally got in the front of the car I had no energy to move. I sat there with a bucket on my lap in case I became sick on the way to the hospital.

"We'll have to try to walk from here," I was told as we drove up the hill to the out-patience area.

I shook my head. "I'm not capable of getting out of the car. How do you expect me to walk the rest of the way up the hill?" I closed my eyes at the thought of me rolling down the hill because my legs had buckled and I had fallen. I could see myself being run over

Ruth Macklin

by the next car coming up the hill to find a park. Or the ambulance screaming up the drive with an emergency patient to hit me.

"Take me to the emergency entrance and get help." After a few grumbles from my husband I was driven up to the emergency entrance where a wheel chair was brought out for me to be taken in to see the doctor.

By the time the car had been parked and Jody carried up to the out-patience where I had been left to wait, a doctor had came out to wheel me in the room. My husband had to wait until he was called into the room because he did not know where I had been taken.

"The results of the test you wife had taken this morning has just reached me. Your wife will have to go into hospital."

Disbelief shone from the eyes of my husband. "She only has gastric. Can't she be given medicine to go home."

"Not possible. You live in a caravan park. Her germ could spread to the rest of the people in the park. That is probably where she caught the germ."

"What is wrong with her?" he was still thinking it was a joke. Why put me in hospital for such a little infection.

"Your wife has two problems. The tests shows she has Hepatitis. The one which is infectious. This is a bad time to get this because she is also pregnant. She could miscarry. Or the baby could be born with defects from the illness."

Ruth Macklin

I was very shocked to hear all the news. Great! I get to spend New Year in hospital. I hated hospitals. I had seen enough of them over the years. What a good start to the new year? Could be a sign I would be spending a lot of time in hospital during the year.

"How long will I be in hospital?" Not that I could run away. I didn't have the energy. I felt it was the best place to be for a few days until I got better.

"That will depend on how long it will take to get you better. The illness has to run its course. We couldn't pick up you had it until we took the blood test. The whites of your eyes didn't go yellow. The blood test is how we picked up what your problem was. You are lucky your daughter, or husband, has not contacted it as well."

Great! Make me feel even worse. I couldn't handle guilt if my daughter caught the disease from me. So I sat quietly as arrangements were made to admit me to the hospital. I was taken to the infectious disease ward. Not that I really cared where I was taken because I was too sick. No good to help my self let alone anyone else. I was helpless. I lay in bed with out complaining as the doctor took more blood for tests. A drip line put in to try to get the fluids back in to the body. I was on the way to becoming dehydrated. It took some time as my veins were hard to find. It was well past visiting hours by the time I have been settled into bed.

My parents arrived the next day from Bundaberg to see me and to take Jody home with them because my husband could not work and look after a small child. When I knew what was to happen I felt at peace to know Jody would be well taken care of while I was sick. I had enough to worry about to get better and try to keep my baby to come without a

miscarriage. Just as well my family worries had been settled because I was there for the

long haul.

I couldn't keep food and water down. Sickness was one problem I had from day one to

the end of each pregnancy. Morning sickness which lasted all day and night. Some times

the drip in my arm would work for a little while then the vein would collapse and the drip

had to be taken out then tried in another place. The amount of times they took blood from

me it was a wonder I had any left as I was not holding enough fluids to rebuild it.

What ever drugs I was given I could not sleep properly. The same as the last sickness

the Avenger of Darkness came to chase me all during the hours of darkness. I tossed and

turned in the bed trying to escape from his clutches. During the night I would bring my

self back to Earth by shouting. The nurses would come running to see what was wrong.

Or the other patients would ring if I kept them awake by yelling. At the time it was

happening I didn't realise I was calling out. It was just a horrible nightmare. My normal

life had been turned upside down. My mind and body were no longer mine. By day the

doctors and nursed poked and prodded. At night I was chased by the Avenger of

Darkness. You are told if you don't eat you will loose weight. For over three months I

could not eat or drink but I never lose weight. I didn't even miscarry. My baby hang on for

dear life. He wanted to live. To come out to see the world.

I was finally well enough to leave the hospital in the beginning of April. I should have

Ruth Macklin

stayed in a few more weeks but my husband had been transferred once again. My legs were so weak when I finally got out of bed. Thinking I would be able to stand on my own my legs but my legs buckled once I put weight on them and the nurses grabbed me before I ended up on the floor. For over a week I was made walk up and down the corridor to try to get the strength back in my legs with a nurse on either side of me holding me up. Finally I got the knack of walking and some energy. In the first week of April I was dress to leave the hospital and taken down to the car in a wheel chair. It felt good to be finally leave the hospital. The first of many problems came when I tried to step up into the caravan at the park. The nurses hadn't tried me on steps. Walking on a flat surface was fine. Stepping up or down was the trouble.

   To get into the caravan I had to sit on the floor, slide backward until I reached the bed where I was able to get on my feet. Going down the steps I had to do the same. The long, slow trip, towing the caravan took it toll and I was exhausted when we finally arrived in Bundaberg. I still hadn't gained the strength in my legs and arms. I had to sit down to cuddle Jody after all those months of missing her. I couldn't walk up the step of the house. There were about fifteen steps. I solved that problem by sitting on the step to gradually move from step to step to get to the top. I lent on a chair to get to my feet. Once on flat floors I could hardly walking.

   After being home for a couple of weeks I soon regained my strength but there were a lot of foods I could not eat. Foods which I once loved to eat either made me sick, or tasted

Ruth Macklin

awful in the mouth. Potato tasted like flour. I used to love seafood but could not eat it. So I just nibbled on foods which I could eat. I was just getting used to handling the steps when it was time to move to our new home. We had to move to Emerald. To live in another caravan park. I was getting sick of living in a caravan. Having to wander around in the night to go to the toilet. Or go over to the shower block to shower, use the toilet and do the washing.

We were only there a week before I got sick once again and had to go into hospital. Once again Jody was taken back to Bundaberg to live until I got better. A week I spent in the Emerald hospital before I was transported by ambulance to Rockhampton to a hospital. The ambulance had to transport a very sick baby to Rockhampton so I was sent along because the doctor in Emerald did not know what to do for me. He wanted me to see a baby specialist. It was a long, slow, rough trip to get to Rockhampton. What ever was wrong with the baby it had to travel at a slow pace.

It was nearly midnight when we reached the hospital and the baby had to be taken to the baby part of the hospital first. I was then taken to the maternity section of the hospital where I was placed in a room on my own away from mothers who had their babies, or waiting to deliver. Once again I was poked, and prodded, to find out what was wrong and how my baby was fairing.

Blood taken again for more tests. Ultrasounds taken to see if my baby was still alive and growing. The worst of the tests the doctors ordered was a liver test. While I lay in the

Ruth Macklin

bed I had local anaesthetic needles in the top of the stomach to make it numb. After a short period the doctor produced this very long needle. My eyes opened wide at the size of it.

"Where am I getting that needle?It looked like something you would use on a horse, or elephant.

"We are going to push the needle into your liver. We need a tiny piece of your liver to do a better test on your liver to tell what to give you to get you better."

"How are you going to do that?"

"Now the area is numb we will push it through here.?he doctor placed his finger on the area where he was going to dig in the needle.

Even though the area had aesthetic I could feel the needle being pushed through the skin to the liver. It felt as though the doctor wanted to go right through me and come out of my back. I had closed my eyes so I could not see what he was doing.

"It will be over in a minute" The sister helped to try to comfort me. To keep me still so the doctor would not miss his mark.

"Finished." He pulled out the long needle. "You can look now." I opened my eyes to see the very small section of liver in the bottom section of the needle. "This will tells us what medication to give you." He went away happy with my pin head size piece of liver. He looked as though he had won first prize in a raffle.

Ruth Macklin

Long Hard Road

After all the results were in the doctor came to see me to tell what he had found.

"At present we can not find any problem with your baby. It is on the small size but that is to be expected from all the sickness you have had. I was happy with that."

"But? There is always a but?" I could see the but written in the look of his eyes.

"Your liver is very badly damaged from all your sickness. Each time you vomit you are doing more damage. From what you say about being sick all through your pregnancy I would suggest you don't get pregnant again. You will have to go on the pill."

I shook my head. "That is not an option. Have tried that but no good to me."

"You should look into some form of birth control. Too many more pregnancies and you will die. You liver will fail."

"I don't want to die so I will look into it once this one is over."

After three weeks in the hospital I was allowed to go home. I walked out of the hospital in the middle of a very cold May afternoon to catch the train to go back to Emerald. My aunt, who put me on the train gave me a lend of a jumper to keep me warm. My feet were frozen by the time the train pulled into the station at Emerald in the early hours of the morning because all I had on my feet were thongs. I felt like a block of ice. My feet didn't have much feeling when I stepped from the train. Our car was parked at the station and I was handed the keys when I got off of the train with a message to tell me when my husband would return from his shift. How I used the brake and clutch on the car

Ruth Macklin

to drive home I don't know. Once in the caravan I turned on the heater, crawled beneath a

heap of blankets and finally fell into a deep sleep once my body warmed.

Ruth Macklin

Chapter Nine

Once I was warm I slept until after midday when hunger and a call of nature woke me. I crawled out of bed, grabbed a change of clothes to have a shower while I was over at the shower block. I didn't want to make two trips in the cold. Didn't want to be as frozen as I was when I stepped from the train carriage.

Life went back to as normal as possible for the next couple of weeks as I tried to rest. I missed not having Jody with me but it was getting close to my delivery time so she stayed in Bundaberg until the new baby was to be born. Even though all the check up went well I had this feeling I would never hold my baby in my arms. Each time I sat to think of how fortunate I was I had not miscarried, my arms were empty. There was no baby for me. There would not be a baby for me. I knew my arms were empty at the moment but the sensation was there telling me this baby would not be held in my arms. It may have been a sign to prepare me for what would come.

Early one morning when I was home on my own I began to get some pains but not very strong. The pains niggled at me all day. They didn't feel like labour pains. I kept doing what I had to do until it was time to go collect my husband when he returned back at the railway station. The pains were getting closer as I drove up to the station to wait. When we arrived back at the caravan one stronger pain hit so I grabbed the bag with a couple of things I had packed during the day. We went up to the hospital.

Lucky for me the doctor was there to see another patient. I was rushed off to the labour delivery room to have my baby. Within half an hour my world had been shattered. The labour pains were gone. The baby was gone. I was left with nothing. No baby!

Not even was I allowed to see him. He was whisked away by the nurse as soon as he was delivered. There was no sound as the baby had been whisked away out of the room.

"Where's my baby? What is wrong with it?I pleaded with the doctor. Hoping against hope my feelings of having no baby to hold was not a warning.

"I'm terribly sorry. Your baby didn't make it. He has been dead for a few days. There was nothing we could do for him."

"At my last check-up he was still alive,I persisted, not wanting to believe what I had been told. I had the feeling I was being lied to. That there was some thing the doctor was not telling me. Felt as though my son had been deformed, or something worse, and they did not want to try to save him. I was never offered a chance to see my baby. I was just empty. Distraught! Why was I being kept in the dark?

I was made ready to go up to the room. A room away from where the babies were kept so I would not hear them cry. So I would not get more upset when I heard other babies cry. The next afternoon I was allowed to go home. Home to make arrangements to have my son buried.

Ruth Macklin

There were only the two of us there, plus the undertaker, to say good bye to a son we never got to see. The unknown body of a baby in a beautiful white coffin with a few flowers on the top. I was devastated. My husband tried to comfort me but I didn't feel as though his heart was involved. As though it was my fault that our son didn't live. There was not a thing I could have done different except not have been in the Townsville caravan park at the time to catch the disease. It probably would have been less traumatic for me if I had miscarried when I had become sick. I may have got better more quickly. And I may not have been left wondering what went wrong. Why did it happen to me? Why was I not given a chance to see my baby? I would have seen for myself what went wrong. May have been upset by seeing why my son did not survive. But I would have known for sure. Not kept wondering why this had happened to this very day.

The only truth was he must have been deceased before I went into labour. When I went for my check-up I also wanted to make plans to have some kind of birth control worked out but it was too late. I was shocked to know I had conceived so soon. The major shock to me was not that I was pregnant again but that I would probably not be around to see my daughter, and the next baby, grow to adults. The specialist had warned me not to try for any more as I would risk my life. I didn't believe in getting rid of the baby so I decided to carry on and face death if that was what was in the future plan for me to live a short life. I would have been in disgrace with my husband if I had wanted to terminate my pregnancy. The doctor gave me medication to try to help me through without being sick too often and kept a check on my liver functions.

Ruth Macklin

In the meantime we had been granted an old house by the railway and we moved in out of the caravan park. We had just got moved in before the baby was born. My son was in a hurry to be born so I had to go to hospital to be given some medication to stop the labour because he was too small to be born. The second time the pains came they stopped on their own then started once again. The doctor decided to put in a drip to help me deliver my baby. I had been in agony all day and nothing happened. The doctor came by to see me before he went home.

"I don't think this baby will be born until tomorrow. I'll come back in the morning to give her some more medication."

That did it! No way was I going to spend any more hours on the hard, labour bed. I had been there long enough. I was hurting from the pains. Was uncomfortable on the hard bed. This baby was going to be born.

"I'll see you in the morning." The doctor told me as he walked out the door.

"No he won't! I won't be here."

"You can't go home," said the nurse. "This baby wants to be born."

"It will be born. I'm not spending all night here." I was determined my baby was going to be born. And now! My determination won out. Within half an hour my son was born. He was small, had yellow jaundice and his breathing was not too well the doctor told me when he returned. My son was put in a humidity crib. My husband was notified at work he has a son but he was not very well. The doctor did not give my son much hope of

Ruth Macklin

making it through the night. The doctor spoke to my husband when he finally arrived at the hospital.

"I think you should have your minister come up to the hospital to have him baptised. He has a lot going against him making it."

My husband walked into the room. I could see he did not like the task he had come to do. He had believed what the doctor had told him. He had no belief our son would make it. He believed our son would die. At first I thought he was mad because he had been called away from work to come to the hospital until the words came rushing out of his mouth.

"Have you see your son?"

"Yes. The doctor wants us to get the minister up here to have him baptised. He said we should do it as he may not survive."

I began shaking my head in the negative. No way was I going to give up on this baby. My other baby I could not have a say. This baby was mine to keep. No way were any of them going to convince me otherwise.

"We have to do it. The doctor said we had to."

"No way! Don't you dare go behind my back and arrange it. I will not have it done. I don't agree with the doctor. He's my son and no way am I giving up on him."

"The doctor said it needs to be done. So he has a name when he dies."

Ruth Macklin

"Neither of you are going to do anything to my baby without my permission. It I let

him be baptised he WILL die. The answer is no. So I was left alone with my decision.

No one bothered me again about having my son baptised." I was allowed to go home after

a couple of days but I visited my son every day. Between us we both showed them we

were the stronger ones. My belief got the both of us through the next few weeks. I bought

material to make nappies for when he came home from the hospital. The nappies I had for

Jody were too big. Philip, as I called my son, could have been wrapped in them to use as a

blanket. I made four nappies from a yard of material and hemmed them on the sewing

matching. The nappies were the size of an extra large handkerchief. It didn't take long

after her came home that Philip was into the right sized nappies. We proved the doctor

and my husband wrong.

This time I made sure I was not going to become pregnant. I went to the specialist to

have tests done and he agreed with the verdict the other doctor had given me. I was never

to get pregnant again. The doctor told me of different birth control methods to be used.

"There is a ring which can be inserted which would be good for you," the Doctor

suggested. "It's very safe."

I laughed at him for that suggestion. "Nope."

"Why not try it?'

"Because it does not work. When I was in having my baby there was a woman who

thought she would be safe wearing it. She produced a baby and the ring came out when

Ruth Macklin

the baby did. I want something permanent."

"Well the only option which is permanent is to cut and tie your tubes. I would not suggest just to tie them because it is not very successful. Sometimes it slips the knot. Putting clamps over the tubes can cause other problems if the body rejects them."

"Fine. I'll go with the cut and tie."

"It is not a decision for you alone. Your husband has to sign that he agrees to you having the operation. You have to think seriously about what you want to do as it can not be undone."

"I would prefer life. I want to be there to see my grandchildren grown. Don't want to be just remembered for the woman who had brought their parent into the world. You set the date and I will be here" The doctor gave me the forms, which I had to fill in and to have signed by my husband. This didn't seem fair to me that I could not make my own decision. That my husband had a say over my body when it came to saving my life. If her did not sign the form I would not be able to have the operation. The decision not to have the operation lay with a man with male pride not because of religious beliefs.

So I went home with my form. On the long trip home I worked out my plan to get the form signed. I had my plan of attack worked out by the time I had arrived. The worse part of the doctor? advice would be tough for him to take. There would have to be no sex six weeks before and after the operation.

When I told him I was advised to have the operation he was not happy. I explained all

Ruth Macklin

the details of what the doctor would have to do to me. He was to sign the form to let me have the operation.

"You'll be a bitch! Spade like a dog. You want me to sign a form for you to become a dog?"

That really hurt! To be classed as a dog. I had not yet explained about the sex bit. This was my turn to hit back. I politely told him the rest of the story without showing I was very hurt by his outburst.

"Well, it is either living with a dog for a wife. Or no sex for the rest of our married life. I don't intend to die just because of your male pride. The decision is up to you. I'll leave the form here in case you decide to sign it. I went to walk off but turned to tell him the rest of the bad news. "There has to be no sex for the next six weeks. There will be none for six weeks after the operation." I could feel the thunder clouds rise as I walked away to see what the children were doing. When I returned to the kitchen to see what he had decided he was not there. The form was signed. I knew where he had gone without being told. He had gone off to the pub to drown his male pride.

On Mother's Day before Philip turned one year old I had been booked into the hospital to have my operation done. I was to have the operation on Monday. The weeks leading up to the operation were very tense. One wrong word and the sparks would fly. I got called all the names my husband could lay his tongue to. They were not very nice names but I just kept my tongue. It was hard to do but there was no way I would do anything to stop

Ruth Macklin

the operation from being done.

I had to suffer a long car drive from Rockhampton to Bundaberg after leaving the hospital because we were on holidays. The clips which had been put in to hold the cut together dug into my flesh with each bump. I had to hold my stomach each time I walked to stop it hurting. The pain was awful. I wasn't given any sympathy. The clips were to be taken out in a week but when the time was up we had to leave to go home. My husband would not take me to the hospital to see if a doctor would take them out before we left to go home.

"You can wait until we get home to go to the doctor. A couple of more days won't hurt."

I wanted to see a doctor because I thought something had gone wrong. Felt there might be an infection but my wishes were over ridden. When I finally made it home to go to the doctor I got told a doctor should have had a look at the wound sooner. The clips were removed but there was a slight infection. With tablets and being able to wash the wound properly now the clips were out it soon got better.

As the six weeks drew to a close the temperature in the atmosphere, not weather wise, had grown into a big thunder storm. He exploded. On returning home from the pub he declared the time was up. He was going to have his rights. I could not stop him. He had signed my stupid form to become a dog. Now it was time he got his payment. He shoved me down on my daughter's bed where I had just changed my son and put back into the

Ruth Macklin

cot. I struggled to try to stop him as there were still a couple of days left of the six weeks to go. I fought but to no avail. With his strength, height, alcohol and sexual frustration I had not hope of saving myself. When he had taken his satisfaction he got up to walk away.

"I'll have you charged with rape because that is what you have just done. I did not consent to that abuse."

"You can't do a thing. I can do what I like in my own home with my wife. Not that you are a wife. You are a nothing."

So he had raped a nothing. It would not have done me much good to bring a report against him. It was just his word against mine. I would have been fawned on by everyone in the close knit area if I had. The law was not for the victim in those days. Now people are listened to when they say they have been assaulted.

The railway did some repairs to the house to make it more liveable. They put new stumps under the house. It was jacked up on packing to hold it there while the new stumps were put in. There was nothing holding the house to the ground. I thought the children would be blown away. Late one afternoon a fierce electrical storm with rain, wind and thunder came rushing toward the town. The dust came first followed by the storm. I sat holding both my children so I could grab them up and jump if the house moved. The house rocked through the storm but it did not fall off the packing. Once the storm had finally finished we went to bed. The lightning show had passed. The thunder

Ruth Macklin

had stopped rebounding around the sky. The rain was lightly falling to wash away the

dust and sand blown in by the strong winds before the storm.

Ruth Macklin

Chapter Ten

My husband met a couple of people at the pub. They were a mysterious pair. A motorbike was usually their transport. No matter how many questions you asked about them the questions were always side stepped or the subject changed. So all the time we knew them we didn't know any more of their family. Or where they had come from before the pair of them arrived at Emerald. They lived in a housing commission house. I don't seem to remember what their surname was. The couple were a very shifty pair. I would have said he was the biker and she was the moll. She tried to look younger by changing her hair from black to blond. Always wore short shorts and very little on the top. Dresses did not cover much. Her skin was well browned and wrinkled from sun-baking. She thought she was sex on legs. Always flaunting what she thought she had. The thing that puzzled me about the couple he didn't seem to worry, or object, to her flaunting her wears. Were they married? What were they hiding? Were they hiding? Maybe if we had stayed longer I may have worked out the puzzle. Or if I would still have been talking to her after the trouble she caused for me.

When the extension to the house had been completed and we had a big, roomy new kitchen and new bathroom my husband decided to have a house warming party. He had invited some of his drinking buddies. There was not a guest who did not drink. Except me. I had seen what could happen to people when too much alcohol had been involved. We had not much furniture as we had not long moved into the house. Some of the people had to sit on the floor.

I didn't want to have the party because I knew who would have to do all the work. Besides looking after two small children all day I had to go out to buy some food and set it out before they arrived. I did some cooking but the rest was cold food. I had worked all day to put on a party I did not want. Could sense there was trouble brewing. Tried to keep a low profile once the children had been put to bed. Had to step over legs of people to get to the room to check they both were still asleep. I finally got told to sit down. By this time everyone were well on their way past caring what happened except for one. One of the other guys warned me what could happen. The only one who still had some of his senses not impaired by alcohol.

The only other female in the group was flaunting her wears. "Watch her! She will have who ever she can get." He must have seen her in action at some other place, or the pub.

She was so drunk she had started hanging on to any guy who would let her. Her..... say husband....didn't seem to try to stop her. He just kept drinking and talking to who ever was sitting next to him. She even began to slobber over my husband but he didn't try to stop her. Maybe even encouraged her to hurt me because since he had used force on me I had shied away from him. Not letting him touch me. Sex went out the door with his act of force. We may have still slept in the same bed but that is all we did. I had no desire for a

repeat performance of his kind of love making. To me it was his way of showing me he

had not forgiving me for having an operation. He wanted a breeder not a wife.

My husband got up to go out side to the toilet. The pair of them had been whispering

before he got up to go. He had not long gone and she followed. Not that her man cared

she had gone outside. Well he did not show any sign of caring where she had gone.

My husband and the moll had stayed out side for a considerable length of time which

looked very suspicious to a drunk person, let alone a sober person. Some of the men must

have felt trouble was brewing because they got up and left. Thanking me for having them

as they walked out the door. The pair of them came back inside as the last person was

leaving. My husband offered to drive him home. The couple left at the same time. No one

offered to help me clean up the mess. The empty beer bottles and the ash trays were

spread all around the lounge room. My nice clean lounge room smelt like a pub. I was

mad about the mess but I set about cleaning away the mess so it would not be there when

the children got out of bed in the morning.

By the time my husband had returned home I had cleaned, tidied and mopped the floor

of the lounge room. I had washed the dirty dishes, dried and put them away. I was

disgusted with the way my so called husband had been acting in front of me, and his work

mates. His actions showed he did not care how he hurt me that there was not an once of

love in him for me. If there ever had been. He was tied to me. His mummy would not

Ruth Macklin

have been happy with him if he had walked out. She would not have been able to see too

much of her grandchildren to be able to spoil them. I should say. Spoil Jody. Because she

did not have a girl of her own to spoil in her own family. The grandson she tolerated but

he never got all the love and spoiling from her which Jody did.

By staying with me he was making my life a living hell. No way could I leave. I would

have had to explain to parents what had happened. I did not want to see my father go to

jail for assault. Or worse. My strength kept me going. He would not make me into a fruit

cake so he could take my children away from me. Like a mother lion. I would stand to

fight and protect my children to the very end.

End. That night I thought my life would end. I don't know how I survived the ordeal. I

was just about to go for a shower before I went to bed to get rid of the smoke and beer

smell from me. The amount of alcohol my husband had consumed during the night I was

worried he may have been picked up for drink driving or had an accident.

"You took a long time. I was beginning to think you may have had an accident." I

didn't yell at him. I was concerned.

"It would suit you if I never came home. You don't want to have anything to do with

me." He was spoiling for a fight.

"Do you blame me. You done the deed."

"You didn't even get mad at what happened with another woman. You didn't care. I

could have had her on the kitchen floor. She was only too willing. At least she wanted

Ruth Macklin

me.' He shouted, his temper rising.

I don't really know what sparked the fuse. I was mad. Blamed alcohol for all the problems in my life. Beer and smokes came before the bills and food. The bill at the pub was paid first when the pay had been collected. He kept some. The rest I had to make stretch to pay the bills, buy food, and clothe the children. More times than I care to remember I lived on bread. Made pickets and scones for me because it was a cheaper option. Food had to be there for him to take to work. I made sure my children were feed properly. He was for himself. When he had spent the money he had kept he came to get more from me. If there was none I had wasted all of his money. The money was never our money.

The next I can remember is I stood with the door of the fridge open. Don't recollect making a move toward the fridge. Was just there with the door open. One after the other I grabbed stubbly of beer from the shelves of the fridge and threw them on the floor, or wall. Where ever they hit. Didn't look to see where they were going. I wanted to destroy the beer. Don't know how he dodged the flying bottles. Next I was being grabbed by the arm to be pulled away from the fridge and the door shut.

"You stupid bitch! What are you trying to do?"

The next my face was stinging. Both cheeks were hit as he kept swinging his hand back and forth. It felt as though he was trying to knock my head from my shoulders. He just kept hitting my face as hard as he could. Temper and alcohol giving him more

Ruth Macklin

strength, and courage, then he would normally have. There was nothing I could do to stop

the barrage of blows to my face. I felt as though I was about to pass out. My knees

buckled and I collapsed on the floor amongst the beer, and broken glass. I had opened my

mouth to tell him to stop when my knees gave way.

"If you were trying to kill me,I whispered as I covered my stinging, sore face with both

my hands waiting for more blows. "You nearly succeeded." I sat there crying waiting for

some response from him. The next noise I heard he had started the car and was driving

out of the yard.

I was left in the middle of the mess. He left me sitting there surrounded with broken

glass and beer. No shoes on my feet to protect my feet when I finally stood up. I had to

slide on the floor until I felt the wall. I could not see. My face had swollen so quickly I

could not open my eyes to see where I was going. I reeked of alcohol now. Once I stood

near the wall I used the wall to guide me to where I wanted to go. My first stop was the

bath room. I stripped off my clothes. Felt for the taps to turn on the shower to wash away

the smell. To try to stop the stinging of my face. Once I felt clean I carefully got out of the

tub to dry myself. I wrapped the towel around my body. Wrung out most of the water of

the face washer to take with me then felt my way along the walls and furniture to make

my way to the bedroom. Thankfully the noise had not woken either of the children. I

could not have been any help to them at the moment. I found my nightdress to put on

before slipping beneath the covers into bed. I covered my face with the wet face washer to

Ruth Macklin

try to relieve the pain, and stinging.

Don't remember going to sleep. Maybe I finally passed out from shock. Did not hear him return to the house. Once his temper had cooled he had returned home. The lights I had left on in the kitchen as I could not find the switch. He must have cleaned up the broken glass and mopped the floor because it was clean in the morning.

The children had woken early and he had gone out to get them something to eat because I had not stirred. I had not heard them make a noise. The first thing I remember is when he came in to wake me. He lifted the face washer from my face to make the light of day wake me. That is when he first seen the damage to my face.

"Shit! What happened to you? Who did it?" I could not see his face. I could not open my eyes to see if it was day, or night. He did sound as though he was shocked.

"You did! If I had not fallen on the floor I would be dead now."

"I don't remember! You sure I did that?"

"Yes."

"You stay in bed. I'll look after the children. Do you want any thing to eat? Or drink?"

"A drink would be good."

That was all I got. Not asked if I wanted to go to the doctor to see what damage had been done. I was never taken to a doctor. The doctor would have had to report the damage to my face to the police. He knew he would have been charged. He knew my father would

Ruth Macklin

have been on our door step within hours and done the same to him. Maybe hurt him

much, much more. He was only thinking of his own skin. I could have died from my

injuries but he didn't care enough to take me to a doctor. I could not take myself because I

could not see. There was no phone. I could not go for help even to the people next door

because I could have ended up worse off than the injuries I all ready had if I wandered in

the wrong direction. Run over by a train.

For one day I was left to lay in bed. I had food and drink brought to me in bed. The

children were kept away from me and not allowed to make any noise. He fed and bathed

them. I had to find my own way through the house to the back door, down three steps,

along a wall to the toilet. I couldn't even see the sunshine when I went down the steps. My

husband went out to buy a record he wanted and gave it to me as a don't tell on me

present. There were a couple of I'm sorry and I don't remember doing it said during the

day.

The next day was a different story. He went off to work and would not be back until

the next night. After the damage he had done to me he could not take a few days off work

to look after me and the children. As blind as I was I had to take care of two young

children. One was still in nappies. I had to take care of them the best way I could. The

doors to the house I kept locked so that either of them would not wander away from the

house. I had to feel to find food for them and hope that I was not giving them something

which may have made them sick, or kill them. Had to try to force one eye open with my

Ruth Macklin

fingers to fill the baby bottle.

The swelling took over a week to go down enough to be able to open my eyes far enough to see. At first my vision was blurred. I wore my sunglasses all day so the children would not be shocked by the sight of the bruising to my face. During all that time I had to keep up with my washing and other work. No way was I going to complain. I had to show I was strong, not a weakling. Was he the kind of person who got his thrill from bashing a woman and pretend he did not do the deed? His hand must have been sore. Or bruised from the hard whacks he dealt to my face. I promised my day would come and he would pay for what he had done to me. What goes around comes around full circle.

One day when I could see enough to drive the car I went to the chemist to get something to bring out the bruising and get rid of the colouring. I asked the chemist man if I could get some cream to bring out bruising.

"What kind of bruising? Where is the bruising?He asked so he could get me the right type of treatment.

I lifted my sunglasses to show him the bruising. The shock which I read in his eyes and on his face told me just what a mess my face was still. He looked as though he wanted to call the police but I don't think he wanted to upset me.

"Have you seen a doctor? Are you feeling sick?"
"No. I haven't been to a doctor. I couldn't see."

"I would advise you to see a doctor." I shook my head to signal no. I knew how much

Ruth Macklin

more trouble would be caused by my attending a doctor to explain how I had gotten my

face bruised so badly. The doctor would have called the police. The police would have

come to ask questions. Once the news leaked out to reach the ears of my father all hell

would have broken out. Within hours my father would have been there to do the same to

my husband. Or he would probably killed him. I didn't want that on my conscious. Both

of the may have ended up in jail for assault. No one would have had jobs to feed their

families. So I stood tall. All alone with my misery. The healing took over a month for all

the bruising to go away but I survived. All the changes in my life, which have been tough

on me, I'm still standing. A bit battled scared but still moving through life fighting to find

peace.

If you are reading this story you may think I was stupid not to have charges laid. You

may think my life was not a very happy one. There were rare times of happiness. The bad

stories are to show you how my character, and strength, were built tough by all the bad

times. There has been years and years of stress in my life which I feel are to blame for a

lot of the illnesses I have had to suffer, and still do, depending on the day and weather.

There is a lot more to come to the building of my character. I believe all these troubles

have been sent my way to test me to see how strong I am that there is a purpose in what

has been planned for me in the future. I also hope this will help others to be strong. To

fight back. To be able to say you are a better person than the one who has assaulted you.

Do not give in. Do not buckle under and say your life is over because of what has

happened to you. If you can tell someone what has happened to help you through the

Ruth Macklin

tough times ahead

Most of the thing which has happened to me over the years has been buried so, so deep, in side of me that I had blocked them out. Over the past few years I have been working to get rid of them because I was told they were holding me back in my life. Now I am doing some de-stressing programs which are bringing the lost memories to the surface. Will explain more as I travel through the rest of the problems which have built me and carried my through to where I am today my dreams for a better future.

Ruth Macklin

Chapter Eleven

After I became better there was a kind of nothing. We each did our own thing.

Pretended we were a family. Sex was something which happened occasionally. Love did

not enter into the equation. When family, or friends were around, we had a kind of truce

where we pretended there were no problems in the marriage. The plan fooled them all. I

don't know if my husband told any of his close friends about what happened. He may

have been too ashamed to tell what he had done to me. Now the time has come to tell the

world. I have been quiet on the matter long enough. I need to get rid of the past to begin a

better life in the future.

In his line of work my husband was responsible for cargo to make sure it reached its

destination without going astray. He didn't do his job well as the temptation to take

parcels he thought he need more than the owner were soon traced to him. He had not been

doing his job properly. Objects started to appear around the house. New objects. I knew

we did not have the money to buy them. I asked where the objects had come from but was

given a cock and bull story never the truth. A movie camera appeared which he used to

take pictures of the family as though he owned it. Not long after that a rifle came home.

Maybe I am lucky to be still alive. Some one up high must have been watching over me.

His parents had arrived to have a holiday with us. The weather had been very wet with

Ruth Macklin

rain pouring down. All the roads into and out of Emerald were closed by flooded rivers. Trains were the only way to get out. It was the worst time for something to go wrong. I had been out somewhere in the car and when I arrived home I knew there had been trouble. His parents were standing on the verandah with the children. Both of his parents had sad, disappointed looks on their faces. At first I thought there had been some kind of argument while I had been gone. Not so lucky.

"What is with the sad faces?I asked, to try to find out what had happened.

"The police have been here. They searched the house. They found a gun and camera. Said they had been stolen. He is being charged now at the police station. He has been given the sack and has a week to get out of the house,explained his mother.

"Great! I leave the house for a few moments and now I don't have a house. No money coming in. He has no job."

"I don't like this either. He should have left things alone. He knew what happened to him the first time," .his mother said.

"We won't be able to stay here. No one will give him a job. Not now he has been sacked for stealing." I was disappointed he could not leave other peoples things alone.

"You will have to move back to Bundy. No one there will know what happened," suggested his father.

"Well I suppose I had better go looking for some boxes to pack all the stuff." What a

Ruth Macklin

time to be packing to move out when the whole area was flooded. Visitors staying in the house. Children to keep occupied. One criminal of a husband to face when he arrived home.

The children could sense something had upset their parents but they were to young to know. I was not there to see how they acted when the police arrived to search the house. I just hope the police were given the articles before they had to make a full scale search through the house. Hope the children were kept away from the proceedings. I never asked because I knew I would not be told the truth. The three of them would have ganged up together to tell me what they thought I should know.

My husband returned home like a dog with its tail between its legs. The searching look from his eyes were waiting for me to haul him over the coals for his light-fingered act once again. No thought had gone into his thinking before he took the articles which did not belong to him. He had just chucked away the best paying job he had ever had. There would be no money coming in to feed and clothe our children. It would take some time to be able, if ever, to get a job where he could be trusted not to run off with something which did not belong to him. I held my tongue. He was being punished for his crime. Now he would have to suffer like I had at his hands. Waiting for me to say something to him for what he had done to the destroy the lives, and trust, of his family.

When most of the packing had been completed his parents boarded a train to take them home to be there for when we arrived. We spent a night in a motel once all our

Ruth Macklin

belongings had been taken from the house and packed on a railway wagon to be

transported to Bundaberg. Our car had to be put on a wagon to be taken to Rockhampton

where it would taken off the train for us to drive the rest of the way to Bundaberg. I was

disgusted with the situation but I held my head high because I was not the one who had

done the crime. I just happened to be married to him.

Exhausted and weary we arrived late and had to spend a few night in the haunted

house until we found somewhere to live before the wagon of furniture arrived. His

mother had been asking around for flats and houses to rent. What we finally had to take

was a small flat in a house which had been converted into four flats. The lino covering the

floor looked as though it had been in the house when it had been built. It was turning up

around the edges with chunks out of it everywhere. It needed a good cleaning. Not that

cleaning would help because the flat was infested with cockroaches. There were that

many cockroaches it is a wonder they did not carry us away while we were asleep. The

flat had a kitchen and lounge room combined, two sort of bedrooms and a bath room and

toilet combined. The washing machine had to be fitted into the bath room for washing the

clothes which had to be carried down steps to be hung on the clothes line out the back of

the building. Living in tents were a castle to living in the flat. There were also fleas in the

ground under the building. I don't know how the owner was allowed to let people live in

such an unhealthy environment.

Moving back to Bundaberg was a big mistake. A mistake with capital letters. He was

Ruth Macklin

back with his old mates who drank to excess. With what little savings we had left after the move my husband kept spending on things he wanted. He wanted gold fish. The tank and fish were bought. An old car was bought. This was suppose to be so he could go out looking for work leaving me with the other car. He was more times running around with his drinking friends, enjoying himself, than worried how his family would live and pay the bills.

Because I complained about what was happening I was a nag. My life got to the stage where I was verbally abused each time he returned home as though everything was my fault because we were in this trouble. I became so stressed out I didn't know whether the children and I would be safe when he returned. To his way of thinking I could not do anything right. Was not a good mother. Was not a good wife. He had been listening to his mother once again. Her wanting to get her hands on Jody.

He finally did get a job but by then it was too late. The money was not there to pay the bills. I was the one who had to face the bill collectors when they came knocking on my door. The last one who came about not paying the car payment was the last straw.

I handed the keys to him. "Here. Take the car. I don't have any money to give you." I was sick of struggling to keep the family afloat on my own. I thought the shock of what had happened to the car would make him see some sense.

The first question when he arrived home from work was, "Where is the car? Have you had an accident with it?" Not that he asked if we were hurt if he thought I had crashed the

Ruth Macklin

car.

I looked him straight in the eyes and told him the plain truth. "This guy came to take it away. The payments were not being paid in full."

"Why were you not paying the payments? You handled the money. They should have been paid."

"What with? There's the rent. Food for you to go to work. Beer money. Smoke money. How much do you think is left to feed and clothe the children?"

"What are you wasting it on? The money I give you should pay for everything."

I smiled. That was the worst thing I could have done. It set him off. I was abused left, right, and centre, for everything he could imagine. I was an unfit mother. The worst wife out. He could do better handling the money. Look after the children better than I could. Plus a lot of other things until he run out of steam. All the time I waited to be on the receiving end of his hand once again. He must have had a feeling he would do it because he down the steps, got in his car and went of for a long time. He either went to lick his wounds or went off to tell mummy what a rotten person I was.

After he went storming off in the car I fed the children, bathed them and put them to bed. I had a snack, cleaned up and went to bed after showering. My nervous system was at a cutting edge. The doctor had given me tablets to try to calm my nerves. I was at the end of the tether. I could take no more of what my husband had been dishing out to me.

Ruth Macklin

Enough was enough. The time had come to take drastic measures. I had to get out of that environment so I did a stupid thing.

I could see no way out for me and the children. Maybe it would be better if I was not there to be the whipping board all the time. So I did what I thought would solve my being mentally abused all the time. I was at the lowest ebb of my life. The tide was about to go out. I climbed back out of bed to go to get a glass of water from the sink. Returned to the bedroom to take about five of the valium tablets from the box which the doctor had given me. I swallowed the lot of them then lay down in the bed. The hope was that I would sleep and never have to face any more abuse from anyone. There would not be anyone for them all to blame, to criticise. I would be gone to a land of peace and tranquillity.

But it didn't happen. I had a very peaceful night's sleep. Didn't hear my husband return to the flat. Never heard a sound until he began shaking me to wake me in the morning. I then knew I was still in the land of misery but something had changed. Sometime during the night a decision had been made. No more was I going to take any more abuse. This was not a suitable environment to raise my children. No way would I ever try to kill myself to make his life happy. He had ruined my life. Now it was his turn to suffer.

As I sat on the side of the bed trying to shake the fog from my brain, I told him, "I'm leaving. I'm taking the children with me. We can't live like this any more."

"You won't be taking the children any where. You can go if you like but they will stay with me. I'll make a better job of looking after them than you have."

Ruth Macklin

"I am leaving. As soon as I can find some where to go we will be gone." My mind was made up and no way was any one going to change it.

"I suppose you are going to stay with your parents? Tell them all sorts of stories to get them to take you in."

"No. I am going to go where I won't be too close to get dragged back to living with you."

"I wouldn't try taking the children if you know what's good for you. You wouldn't have the guts to leave."

He went off to work thinking the discussion had been solved. Thinking he had bluffed me into his way of thinking. I had a small amount of money I had been saving. Sold some coins I had been given a long time ago. Used that money to put fifty cent places on horses and soon I had the money I needed. I bought a very large suitcase in which I started packing thing which I wanted to take with me. Clothing I left to the last minute when I had purchased my bus ticket to take me away. I had inquired how much I would need for the bus ticket and save a little extra money for food to get me to my destination. It was a very big step I had decided to take. A couple of days before I went to buy my bus ticket I began to pack the clothes I wanted to take with me in the suitcase and a bag.

"You still think you are leaving,my husband jeered, when he looked at the packed suitcase.

"Yep! Any day now. You will have your chance to prove you are a much better parent

Ruth Macklin

than I am. We'll see how you manage."

"You wouldn't walk out without the children."

"You just wait and see."

I went to the travel agent to purchase my ticket during the day ready to leave town. Went to bed as though I had no plans of going anywhere. Early next morning I got out of bed to have a drink and a snack then went down the street to the phone box to ring for a taxi to take me to where I was to catch the bus. My luggage was waiting at the door for the taxi to arrive when my husband crawled out of bed.

"Where do you think you're going? I have to get ready for work. Who do you think is going to look after the children?"

"I'm leaving! I told you I was. You now have what you wished for. The children are all yours." The taxi man came up the steps to take down my luggage. I kissed both the children good bye then walked down the steps to the taxi with a heavy heart. Crying deep inside.

I had tears in my eyes for the children I was about to leave behind. I loved them dearly but I had no way of knowing what lay ahead of me once I got off the bus at the end of my journey. I didn't know if I would have a place to sleep. If I would have had more money I would have taken my children with me. I had to get as far away as possible so I would not be harassed into returning to the environment I had escaped from. Everyone would have wanted an explanation why I had run away without telling anyone why I had to do it. That

Ruth Macklin

would be setting a cat among a flock of pigeons. The whole story would have had to

come out. Even though I wanted to catch the next bus back to Bundaberg from Brisbane I

made myself hop on the connection bus to continue on my way.

I finally stepped of the bus in Melbourne. Tired and in need of a bath after days of

continuous travelling I just wanted to find somewhere to go to sleep. To sleep in a bed

which did not move. Not feel the vibration of the engine of the bus as we travelled day,

and night, to reach our destination. I was pleased to get off the bus for the last time.

My plan was not without error. I didn't know the day I arrived would be a holiday in

Melbourne. Nearly every place was closed. Finding my luggage when it was unloaded

from the bus, I made for the taxi rank to get taken to the address which I had where I

knew I would be able to get help. The taxi driver took me to the address but the building

was closed. Luck was with me. The driver could see I needed help. He knew of the person

who I had put my faith in to help me. The driver stayed with me until the man arrived.

While I explained to the Father my predicament another car arrived with people in to

see him. The Father had rang the family to come to his office. Once I had been checked

out to the Father's satisfaction that I was not a crook. Or a killer. Or something worse.

The man came in to the office and I was introduced to him. There entailed a short

discussion to see if I would be suitable to be employed to be a housekeeper to the man

and his three small children. Their housekeeper had walked out and the children had no

one to be there for them while the father worked. After handshakes I found myself and luggage bundled into the car to be taken to meet the grandparents of the children then we went to their home where I was given a room of my own.

I was made to feel at home from the very beginning. My first job was to unpack a change of clothes and head for a log shower to wash away the grime, and tiredness, from my long trip. The shower seemed to wash away some of my troubles and felt a different person about to start a new life. I had a job and somewhere to live. At least I didn't have to sleep out on the street because that is what I probably would have had to do if not for the help of the kind and caring taxi driver.

Ruth Macklin

Chapter Twelve

Thought everything would run smoothly for me. For the first couple of days everything worked well then toward the end of the next week I was kept busy. Michelle, Leanne and Nicole went down with the measles, one after the other. Most of the day was spent keeping them cool. Beds clean. Making sure each of them had a bucket in which to be sick. This was a busy time until the worst of the sickness had passed. Maybe this was a test to see if I was capable of looking after three girls and a home. Whether I could be trusted to stick to the job and not walk out on them when they were really in need.

Someone must have listed me as a missing person because a few weeks after I had been working a police officer arrived at the door looking for me. He came to check out that I was safe. That I was living there on my own free will. I had left a few false ideas to where I had thoughts of going. What I might like to do.

"I have no intention returning to my husband,I told the policeman. □ ou can send word to let my family know I am safe but not where I live. I don't want to be hassled."

The policeman agreed not to divulge my whereabouts to anyone. I had assured him I was safe and knew what I was doing. I could have explained all the reasons why I had left but I would not be at the other end to stop any trouble. I didn't want to be dragged back to give evidence if the police got too involved. A clean break. I missed my children and cried most nights I went to bed. I had to make a new life so one day I could have my

children with me. When their father realised he was not as capable, and smart, as he kept

thinking he was. He may have been older than me but he was not wiser.

He proved he was not wiser. Had to run to his mummy to help with the children and a

place to live once he finally realised what a mess he had put his family in. He finally

found an address where to send letters to me pleading for me to return for the sake of the

children. The letters were passed on to me. The letters was very upsetting to hear how my

children were taking my disappearance. But I had to be strong. My life would have been a

living hell if I had returned to try to continue as a family. I would have been picked on, or

questioned, by all relations why I had felt the need to leave. His parents would have been

the worst. Especially his mother because she would not have believed what her son was

capable of doing.

Then came his trump card. The cruel plan he had set in motion. The pack of lies he

had spun to get his own way. To hit back for the slack he was probably getting from all

the family. Not having the freedom he had been used to having for most of our time

together. He thought I would come rushing home without checking out to see if his story

was true.

I received a phone call late one afternoon form the Father who had helped me.   " I

received a phone call from your husband. I'm afraid it is bad news. He told me to let you

know your daughter Jody was hit by a car and killed on her way home from school. I'm

Ruth Macklin

sorry to have to be the one to tell you the news."

I was shocked. Didn't know what to say. "Did he say anything else about the accident? What time it happened? Where she was when it happened? Did she make it to the hospital?" The tears were streaming down my face because I was not there to save her. To protect her from being hurt.

"No," he didn't tell me too much. He left a number where you can reach him."

"Thank you for passing on the message, Father."

"Sorry this call had to bring you bad news."

I knew not to ring the number I had been given because my husband, or his mother, would have answered the phone. I rang some family members to ask if there had been an accident that afternoon. To get them to check out the truth of the phone call. I had this feeling that something was not right. If it was true why had the police not been the ones to tell me of the news. Why had my estranged husband been the one to make the call? I left a number where I could be reached if the story was true. But the story was not true! He had thought up this cruel, sick joke, using our daughter as bait to lure me back to Bundaberg. It did but not when he was expecting me to return.

After that lie which I had not let anyone know about I started to make plans to go get my two children. I had been hearing rumours about how the children were being treated. How Philip was being made to feel the black sheep of the family. So I rang my parents once my plans had been made to return to Bundaberg for a short trip. A great aunt of the

Ruth Macklin

girls had been organised to come to be at the house while I was away. I hopped a bus with enough clothes to last a few days. It was going to be a swift trip. I would be on the move all the time. Had no idea what I was going to do once I got to the other end.

My cousin waited for me at the bus stop when I arrived in the early morning and took me to her place. My parents arrived not long after from Sarina where they lived. We had to be careful we were not caught in town, or caught at what we were about to do. I could not beard the lion in her den to tell her I had come for my children. I would have been stopped. We went to a place where I was given some very good advice, and help. I am very grateful to the couple of elderly ladies who gave me such good advice in my hour of need. They were there to give advice and thankful they listened to me.

Not long after our discussion I was driven up to the school where I knew Jody went to school. I went to the principle to tell him I wanted my daughter. I was there to pick her up to take with me. Jody was sent for and she came into the office and came straight to me.

"Mummy! When did you come home. Where are we going?" She was very excited to see me. Even more excited when she believed we were playing a trick on her father.

"You can go with your mother now. Don't forget to collect your school bag on your way out."

Jody chattered away as we made our way to get her school bag and out to the car. "Which kindy is Philip at? I want to surprise him too."

Jody showed us where to collect Philip. There were not too many questions asked

Ruth Macklin

because I had Jody with me and Philip did remember me, which I was not sure he would. We went to where my parents were waiting for us. There was another hitch in the plan. The children had no clothes. Jody could not go wearing her school uniform in case we were stopped during our travels.

Clothes were borrowed from a family friend who had small children around the same age. Not long after the children were fixed for clothes we were bundled in my parents car and driven to Maryborough to catch the bus. I was advised not to wait to catch a bus from Bundaberg.

While we made our escape to Maryborough my cousin went around to the grandparents house to tell them not to go to collect the children from school, or kindergarten, because I had returned to collect my children and take them away with me. The grandparents had to be told what had happened so there would not be a scare when they found out the children were not where they were suppose to be.

Once we arrived at Maryborough, tickets were purchased for Jody and Philip as well as my seat had to be booked because the ticket I had was an open one. There was no telling how long I would take to collect the children. Whether I could get them without too much hassle. I know the way I got them back was under handed but I would no longer have to worry each day how they were both being treated. I had no choice in the decision because I knew their father would put up every road block to stop me having them just to spite me.

Ruth Macklin

We went to stay with my aunt and uncle until it was time to catch the bus. Later that

night we went to catch the bus to get back to Melbourne. All I seemed to have done since

I let Melbourne was sit in a bus, or a car, to achieve what I had set out to do. Both of the

children thought it was a kind of an adventure. They were going to see all these new

places, and people. There would be a new home for them and other children for the to

play with. The bus was an express so we seemed to keep moving with a few stops along

the way. Some time during the trip Jody became bus sick and vomited all over her

clothes. I had to try to clean he as best as I could because I could not get to my bag to find

any more. So the rest of the trip was a bit smelly. No one knew when I would be returning

home to Melbourne. With the last of my money we caught a taxi to take us home.

Luckily for us some one was home to let us in. The great aunt and the three girls were

there to welcome us home. Everyone was excited to see me return. I think they had a

feeling I might not return. Or I would be away for a long time getting my children from

their father. Once the greetings and introductions were over the three of us went to have a

bath to get clean. To try to wake up from three days of non stop travelling. We were all

sitting in the lounge room when Robert returned home from where he had been. It was

Good Friday. He was thrilled to see I had returned so quickly. We settled in to be like a

family.

Once my one year of separation had come around I went to file for a divorce. So the

divorce would not drag on for years with a long custody battle, I let the lawyer convince

Ruth Macklin

me to sue for non comparability. I did not sue for mental and physical abuse like I wanted

to do. As I had not gone to the doctor and police were not involved it would have been

my word against his. I would have had to return to Queensland to fight the suit. It was

quicker and cleaner not to drag out our dirty washing in public for all family and friends

to know. After all he had done to me I was still trying to save his rotten hide. But I had

won. I was free from him. I had my children. Even thought he was suppose to send

twenty dollars per week to the court for the upkeep of the children I never received a cent

from him. He did not even fight for visiting rights. Maybe he was pleased to get rid of

them to have his freedom to do as he pleased.

Only once I returned to the haunted house to collect all my belongings which I had left

behind. I had given the lawyer a list of what I owned before we were married. The items

had to be there when I went to collect them from his mother. I should have worn them I

had thought about leaving. Maybe things could have been sorted out. I had taken Jody,

Philip, Michelle, Leanne and Nicole with me on the trip to Queensland. We flew up to

Mackay then drove to Bundaberg to collect all my things and for the children to see their

grandparents. Their father was not at home at the time. I believe he knew we were coming

but he did not stay to see his children. It would have been too hard for him to see them for

a few minutes and have them taken away again. Making out it was all my fault once

again. Some time would have been better than no time at all. I had paid out all the money

for us to go to see them but that was not seen as a sacrifice on my part. No one seemed to

appreciate I had made an attempt to bring the children all the way to see them.

Ruth Macklin

The both children felt snubbed. Their father did not want to see them. It hurt them that they had come to visit but they were not welcome. We were all outcasts. So I did not attempt at that stage to keep in contact for the children's sake. They put that life behind them and settled into life in Melbourne. We all kept busy so no one would get home sick for a family who no longer cared.

As a family we went to different places together. The zoo. Visiting family. On picnics. I even learnt to drive through all the Melbourne traffic. Never was I going to drive when I first had seen all the roads, cars and trucks. Even had to dodge around trams. I had not seen so much traffic as most of my life had been lived in the country and a few bigger towns. Most of these I had live in or passed through during my growing years. They did not scare me. Cars coming at me from all directions was another thing. I was offered the car to drive but I had declined. Until one day we had gone to Ballarat for the day. A work mate who did shows as a side line was at Ballarat doing a show. Some how there happened to be one too many cars and not enough drivers.

"I don't know how we are going to get all the trucks home,'" complained David. "We are one driver done. One of the helpers got sick."

"I'll drive it back for you," offered Robert, trying to be helpful. Other wise someone would have had to be brought back to drive the other truck home.

"Who's going to drive your car home? You can't leave your family here until you come back."

Ruth Macklin

"Ruth can drive. She can drive my car back to your place," was Robert's suggestion.

"Oh, no I can't. I've never driven you car. I won't drive on roads I don't know. Count me out. No way did I want to drive all those hours on roads I had never driven on. What happened if I got lost? Got cut off with traffic. Might have been okay in the daylight. It would be dark before we got back to Melbourne. I would not be able to find the land marks."

With some verbal arm twisting I found myself behind the steering wheel of the family car. I was driving on strange roads in the dark sandwiched between trucks so I would not get lost and they would have to come back looking for me. Lucky the children had dozed off so I could concentrate on the road, and the holiday traffic moving back into the city.

Finally we arrived at our destination where the trucks had to be stored in Dave's yard. It was a pleasure to get out of the driving seat of the car. My legs shook as I got out of the car. It was a lesson. If you fall off a horse you should get back on to ride it once again otherwise you will never ride again. From that day on I began to drive around close to home. Then another day I went to visit family on the other side of the city. The drive there took us half an hour. On the way home, with a lot of wrong turns and a round about way I took two hours for a trip which should have taken half an hour. But I learnt from my mistakes. The only way to find your way is to get lost and you have to concentrate on land marks which will help you find the way you are suppose to be going. By trial and error, I soon learnt my way around a fair few of the suburbs and became game enough to

Ruth Macklin

drive in the main part of the city. I didn't even have a fight with a tram for the road.

All I needed was a gentle push to get me behind the wheel of the car. Now I had freedom to get around the area to do the shopping and go to places when time permitted. I even fought my way through show day traffic to get to the show on show day holiday. What a bad day to go to the Melbourne show. I went to the pavilion to get each of the five children a show bag. Big mistake! It was shoulder to shoulder people to get through the pavilion. You stopped to look and you got shoved to move on. In desperation, I finally grabbed some show bags with the hope the children would like them. Didn't have much chance to ask what the bags contained.

"I'll have that one,I pointed at the board and kept pointing until I had the required amount. Then I had to shove my way out of there with the bags hoping I still had them when I reached the outside.

Once I had bought all the items I wanted for the children I walked around the ground until I found the exit near where I entered the show grounds, slowly dragging my feet to make my way back to the car. I thought my troubles were over once I made it safely out of the grounds but I was mistaken. When I went around the side of the car to load in all the bags I found I had a flat tyre. I kicked the shoes from my tired feet and set about getting the jack and spare tyre out of the back to change the tyre. Luckily the spare was ready to put on, not flat. I was pleased when the tyre was fixed so I could go home to have a refreshing shower and rest my aching feet.

Ruth Macklin

The children were told I was to have the day off because I had been working hard. I needed some time to myself for a few hours. If they had known I had planned to go to the show they would all have wanted to go with me and it would have cost more money. I received cuddles from them all when I arrived home with the show bags.

Ruth Macklin

Chapter Thirteen

We went everywhere as a whole family. Not you and your children have to stay at home because I need to take my children out. Two families working together as one. No one got treated differently to the other. We went fishing. Picnics out at a river where it was safe for everyone to swim. One Sunday we left early with another family to go out to the river to have the whole day out. We took a picnic lunch with us. The place was peaceful with the sound of the rushing water and the birds singing in the trees. It felt as though I was living back out in the country but we were only a few kilometres from town. The day had been made to relax and restore calmness to the body and the spirit.

The day was drawing to a close when we arrived home. The other lady wanted to go to church so I changed and went with her. Her husband and Robert looked after the children while we went. There was nothing to worry about when we left the house. The children were all taking turns in the bath to get clean from their day out and be in their pyjamas by the time I returned to have dinner before going to bed.

As I turned the car into our street it was alight with flashing red lights. Two fire trucks were parked in front of the house. Men in uniforms rushing in and out of the house. There was no sign of smoke coming from the house. Or any other house either side of the house. I had to find room to park the car in the street out of the way. I rushed toward the house to find out what had happened while I was gone.

Ruth Macklin

Some of the children came rushing out of the front door to meet us. They were all

excited about what was happening and all tried to tell us the news at the same time.

"Nicole's stuck in the bath! She can't get out! We had to call the fire brigade."

"Why can't Nicole get out of the bath?" I knew the bathroom and didn't think anything

in there was dangerous enough for her to get stuck.

"Her fingers are stuck in the plug hole. The water sucked them down." Shaking my

head is disbelief I walked into the house and straight into the bathroom. Sure enough.

There   sat Nicole in the bath with a towel wrapped around her naked body with three of

her fingers stuck down the holes in the drain. As she had taken the plug out to let the

water run down the drain, she had not been quick enough to get her fingers out of the

way. The strong suction of the water sucked her small fingers into the round holes in the

drain.

Nicole calmly sat there waiting for someone to get her free. She looked as though she

had been crying at first but with all these strange people in her bathroom must have

calmed her. Some firemen were in the bathroom watching she didn't get any more hurt

than she was. Robert and other firemen were under the house trying to dismantle the

plumbing to be able to get the plug out of the bath tub so the firemen could work to get

her fingers out of the plug.

Finally the plug was released to be able to be pulled from the hole in the bath. A

fireman got Nicole to stand up while he juggled the drain out. I wrapped the towel more secure around her now shivering body because it had been getting cold while she sat there partially wrapped in the towel. A fireman carried Nicole out to the kitchen and set down on the table. A vice was then set up on the kitchen table to place the brass drain in to hold it still while the firemen worked on getting the fingers from the holes.

Because the job had taken so long to get Nicole out of the bath the big boss fire chief from Melbourne City fire station came out to see what was keeping the two brigades busy for so long. He walked into the kitchen to find Nicole on the table with a fireman with a wire thin cutting file cutting his way around the spikes which released two of her fingers. A third one was still stuck in the middle hole when her hand could be moved away from the drain. Then that had to be worked on carefully so as not to cut her finger as the ring was cut off. After three hours of working to free her fingers Nicole was finally released of the last piece of the drain without even a scratch to show what she had done. The drain was put back in the hole in the bath so the rest of the family could have their bath. A new improved piece had to be put in the next day so no more fingers would be sucked down the drain. Nicole had been the third child that week the fire brigade had attended. One was in a flat in a high rise building. The house was very quiet after everyone had left. The drama over and past time to go to bed.

What started out to be a relaxing day ended with a lot of drama. The men were worried they would get blamed for what happened. Thought I would say they were not looking after the children properly. But an accident is an accident. It could have been any one of

Ruth Macklin

the children with small enough fingers to be sucked down the hole. The design of the round holes of the drain and the strong suction as the water rushed out of the bath were to blame. Now most drain holes are made different to stop fingers going down with the water. Only the older home with the old drains still in them would have to be watched. She had not been sitting there trying to put her fingers down the hole. No amount of lubrication would let the fingers slip back up the way they had gone down.

With a family of five small children there were always small things going wrong. Like the day the children were riding up and down the street to go to the park at the end of the street. Leanne was speeding up the footpath to get somewhere in a hurry. She came to a sudden stop. She could not have been watching where she was headed. A planted stop sign jumped out to get her. Meaning she ran into the stop sign on her bike. Hit her forehead on the steel pole. By the time she had made it back to the house she had a big lump on her forehead. After a little cry and a lot of sympathy she was back out on the bike. It is still a joke in the family about the day a stop sign jumped out and hit Leanne. Not her who ran into the stop sign.

After I had my papers to say I was now a free from my marriage I knew I would no longer be pestered to go back to a life where I would probable not have been still here to tell my story. I could do as I pleased. We were one big happy family. Once Robert had made a trip up to Sarina on a holiday with a mate he came back to say he would like to move to Queensland. The weather was better. So plans were put into action about

Ruth Macklin

moving. There was a big discussion between us and we decided to marry and keep the lot of us together as we had grown as a family. It would have hurt the children to have been pulled apart. To have to get used to knew parents all over again.

Robert's three girls, Michelle, Leanne and Nicole lost their birth mother at a very early age because she died. My children, Jody and Philip lost their father through divorce. We had been living separate in the house but we treated everyone as a daughter, or son. Everyone never got classed as being better than the other like in some two families joining to become one. We all had to share with each other. In January 1978 we became married in the backyard at our home. Family and friends were invited by word of mouth. Others in the street just dropped in to wish us well. It was a very friendly street where everyone came to each others aid, or helped where they could.

My mother made four long dresses for the girls to wear to the wedding and Philip had a little blue suit. The dresses were a different colour for each girl. My parents came down to Melbourne for the wedding and they were the witnesses at the ceremony. I did most of the food for the wedding. Even made the wedding cake. The icing was a bit hard because I had trouble to get it to set in the hot weather but it done the job. The cake was moist and fruity to make up for the bad icing. There was a ride from one of Robert's mates who done the show circuit for the children to have rides on to keep them amused.

Toward the end of the year I had to start sorting out all the items in the house and pack them up ready for the shift to Queensland. In the new year before the start of the new

Ruth Macklin

school year the children and I moved to Sarina to wait for the house to be sold. We stayed with my parents. The children began school as we waited for the sale of the house. After Easter the house finally sold. Robert and a family friend transported the packed boxes, and furniture, to store under his house in Brisbane, where it stayed until it was to be brought through to the house. The last load they brought all the way to Sarina to store under my parents house until we found a house to buy.

While we were staying with my parents my mother and I went to play bingo when the children were at school. When we arrived home I got a phone call to say Leanne had been taken to the doctor from school. She was waiting at the doctors for me. It seems at lunch she was playing in the school yard jumping from one car tyre to another which had been set in place with cement, she missed her footing and fell on to the cement. Ouch! One very badly broken forearm. A piece of the broken bone had pierced the skin. Leanne was more worried about getting into trouble for breaking her arm than worried about the pain.

How was she going to explain to her father she had broken her arm. At least her father was too far away to yell at anyone when he was phoned to tell him the news. So it was a trip to the hospital in Mackay where it was x-rayed, pulled back into place and a plaster cast put on. Leanne had to return to the hospital the next day to have it checked to see if it had swollen during the night making the cast too tight. She had to have the cast on until the break healed. A forty minute drive each way to get to the hospital in Mackay. She knew to keep off of the tyers from then on.

Ruth Macklin

The first week Robert arrived he found a job of shovelling coal from rail wagons to clean them. When we had time to look we found an old, small house, in which to live. It needed some work done on it. My father and a few other friends helped to do some of the immediate alterations to make more room so we would not be squashed in like sardines.

The kitchen if that was what it could be called was a pocket size area with a very dirty electric stove, a sink and a very old cupboard with stain glass set in the two top doors. There was a pantry built into the wall. No wall closed it off to make it a room. Once we would have put in a fridge there would have been no room left to fit in a table to hold seven people. In the house section were two rooms, a large lounge room and a sleep-out. Down a couple of steps were the bathroom, toilet, laundry and a car shed which had all been added to the house after it had been moved to where it now stood. Luckily it was all cemented.

Timber walls in the shed were torn away to line the wall to make the shed into a new kitchen. The timber was replaced with sheets of white Masonite to line the walls and ceiling. A new gas stove was bought to put in the new kitchen. Another sink as well. My father made this never to be broken table to sit lots of people. The legs and the top to hold the wood were made of box steel and welded together, not bolted. Over the steel was placed a piece of board with a piece of laminate on the top with a strip of metal edging around the edge. The table took a couple of strong people just to move it.

Glass and wood sliding doors replaced the roller door to make it look more like it was

Ruth Macklin

a part of the house, not a kitchen in a shed. Windows had also been put in at one end and

two sets on one side. More cupboards were bought to fill in the large area and new chairs

to fill the length and ends of the table. When the renovations were all completed we

moved in. The old kitchen had been pulled apart to make that into a bedroom. A partition

and door were added to make it more of a room not an open area. One of my cousins

came to Sarina for a holiday and built a wardrobe and duchess into the main bedroom. It

went the whole length of the wall and a couple of feet from the ceiling. There were two

sets of double wardrobe doors, draws down the middle section, an open area for a mirror

and place to put combs, as well as other items. Right across the top were sliding doors.

We had plenty of room.

After awhile Robert got a job of driving the railway car where he took notices out to

the workers to tell them when they were needed to go to work. Drive all over the country

side to get train crews to their train. It was back to shift work once again. I had been used

to normal hours for a few years. Now it was back to different shifts. Never knew when

Robert would be called into work if someone went off sick and he would have to do a

twelve hour shift. Trying to sleep with a house full of children when they were home

from school was not good when Robert had to sleep during the day. The hard part was
trying to keep them from making too much noise.

Once we were settled into the house our lives were kept busy with work and children.

Driving Robert to and from work. Driving children to school until they were old enough

to walk the short distance to make it on their own. Then my parents moved from railway hill on the south side to be closer to the shops. They were about half way between us and

the school. Things were working smoothly until everyone got over worked, and over

tired, with a few children problems thrown in as they grew older.

Philip had a problem with school. He either didn't turn up. Ran away. Or got into a lot

of trouble. He had a good brain for trouble and doing thing he wanted to do but learning

at school was not one of his strong points. I never knew what to expect next which didn't

help the nerves, and stress level, because I was getting complaints from everyone about

him.

"You should do this. You should do that. Why don't you make sure he listens to you?

You should be making sure he does his homework. He wants a good belting. Stand over

him to make him do as he is told," I had all these voices running around in my head from

all these people trying to tell me how to control a child who had a rough start in life. He

had to fight to get recognition from his father's parents from baby on ward. With four

girls older than him he was still fighting to get to the top of the hill.

I did the rounds of the doctors with him to try to sort out his problem but not much

seemed to help. He was just with the wrong people who wanted to run wild. I never knew

what to expect next. He would disappear for days on end then return some times of his

own free will other times with the police. I just had to say , "No news is good news,"

when he did his disappearing act because if he didn't want to be found you could not find

him. Only hear where he had been.

Ruth Macklin

Then the crunch came. He had to face the children's court for stealing. That was the end. I could not see a way of getting through to him. Philip was taken into care and sent off to a foster home. He stayed there for awhile going to a different school and we would go to visit when we were told we could. But that did not last for long before he decided to go walk about. He was missing for about a week before he finally turned up back at home. There were many kilometres from where he was put to our home. Never found out which way he travelled to reach Sarina. Whether he walked across country or went into Mackay and back out to Sarina.

This time he was put in a detention home in Townsville where he had to stay until he calmed down. It was a hard decision to have to give the care of your child to strangers to see if they could do a better job at caring for him than you could. I didn't want him to keep travelling down the same road which his father had done. Temper was one of his main problems. Highly strung. His way was the right way. The doctors tell you to keep him away from sugar and other products. If he could not get them given to him he would sneak them out of the cupboard, or go steal them from somewhere. There was not way of stopping him once he had made up his mind. I could talk quietly, yell until I was blue in the face but it made no difference. Five seconds later he would be doing the same thing.

Ruth Macklin

Chapter Fourteen

Life was always busy. There was never dull moments as the children grew older. They all had their different wants and needs.

Different friends and things to do. Places to go. Robert had joined different clubs. We helped raise money for the ambulance centre by selling raffle tickets plus ham and chicken raffles at the hotel on a Sunday. Helping with the bingo. All time consuming work. Robert was also a member of a club which met every Friday night. At some stage I had been given the job to supply their nibbles which they consumed during the night with their alcohol. I was dragged to the women's side of the club where we did things to raise money for the club.

Most of the women were older and had all the ideas but few of them wanted to do the hard work to pull the ideas together. Some didn't have cars. I felt I had to carry a lot of the running around to get items together for the Hoys they wanted to have. Hoy is like bingo but played with thirteen cards per hand rather than fifteen numbers like bingo. Prizes were food items. A mini cent sale consisted of prizes like hand towels, face washers, plastic wear, food, home made cakes. Then there had to be sandwiches for morning, or afternoon tea, depending on what time of the day the hoy was held. All this extra was expected of you besides looking after a husband, five children and keeping the house cleaned, washing done, food cooked and find time to sleep. The working hours in each day were very long. Most days I needed more hours to get all the work done.

As the months passed it seemed to me as though we met as husband and wife while passing through a revolving door. One coming in and the other going out. Like being on a merry-go-round. You caught a bit of sleep when you could. Dragging me in all different directions. I wanted to get off but I did not see a way of doing it so I kept trudging alone. Kept my cool when I could have let off a full head of steam. I could of packed up and went of for a good holiday to relax the nerves and rest the body as well as the mind. But alas! I had to keep going and not complain only grumble to myself when no one was listening.

One afternoon when every member had plans for the afternoon I went to a cent sale with an old lady friend called Kath. It was a very peaceful afternoon where I could sit and relax for a few hours without someone wanting me to do something for someone. Robert had offered to take a friend back to his place of work at the other side of the Sarina Range. Philip and Nicole wanted to go for the drive. Kath's husband Wally went with Robert and the children for a change of scenery from sitting at home all the time.

I had not long walked in the door of the house after leaving Kath at her home when the phone rang. I had the feeling during the afternoon something was going to happen. Something bad. The rest of the children were with friends. I was the only one home. A shiver ran down my spine as I picked up the receiver.

Ruth Macklin

"This is the Sarina police. Does your husband own a brown Valiant sedan?"

"Yes. Hoping he had not drank with the friend and been caught for drink driving.

"The car has been involved in a single vehicle accident on the top of the range. We have just been advised about the accident."

"Are any of them hurt?"

"We don't know. We are headed out to the accident scene now. Could you meet us out there?"

"Sure! I'll leave now," I dropped the receiver then picked it up again to let my parents know where I was going for them to tell the other children when they returned home. I also scribbled a hasty note to leave on the table then took off in the car for the accident scene. Praying everyone was alive and not badly hurt.

At any other time I hated driving up and down the Sarina Range. Always took the drive slow. Watched out for cars coming from the other way on the very sharp bends. Didn't want to be hit and pushed over the side of the range never to be found among the thick trees until it was too late. Didn't want to be left there for the animals to feed on. I always keep my eyes focused on the road ahead. But that night I went up the range as fast as possible. I arrived at the accident scene moments before the police car. I got out of the car but there were no one to be found. Against the steep bank to the inside of the road was the car on its side. It was buckled and bent out of shape. The windscreen broken. The car had gone end over end before ending on its side against the bank.

Ruth Macklin

"Is this your husband's car?" I was asked.

"Yes. But where are they?"

"We got another call on the way out here to say they were taken by a semi driver to the ambulance station."

"Are they all okay?"

"We don't know. Do you give us permission to have the vehicle towed out of the way?" I agreed they could do what they like with the crumbled mess. It would never be driven again. It would be scrap metal.

"Is there any more you want to know? I want to find my family." The police didn't need me there so I turned the car around as the police watched for traffic coming down the range. I headed back down the range to try to track down my family. The fast drive up and down the range were completed but I don't remember much about the trip. The brain seemed to have shut out the drive once I had seen the mess of the car body. I couldn't see how they would have made it out without being badly hurt. There were only two seat belts in the car. One for the driver and the passenger. None for the rest of the passengers. A time before they were made legal.

I screeched to a stop at the ambulance station. Jumped out of the car. Ran into the building to try to get some information thinking my family may have been transported straight through to the Mackay hospital. The four of them had been rushed up to the Sarina hospital to be checked out before being transported. I raced back out to the car to

Ruth Macklin

go to the hospital a few streets away. Lucky no one was in the way as I drove into the hospital parking lot. For a change I had my choice of parking spaces. There were no other car there. Racing up the rest of the hill to the entrance to the hospital and in the door. I came to a sudden stop. There on a chair sat my son. He was all in one piece except for a blood nose. I nearly collapsed but I had to hold it together. My family needed me to stay strong. I was sitting with my arm around Philip listening to him tell me what happened when the nursing sister found me.

"It was dark. I couldn't see. I found the torch and shone it around the car. When I felt the car begin to roll I braced my feet against one door and held on to the handle on the other. Philip tried to explain all the things which had happened at the time of the crash. ? he car was in the middle of the road. I climbed out of the car with the torch to stop anyone for help. Flagged down a truck coming down the hill. He helped get everyone out of the car. Then he drove us to the ambulance station."

"You did a good job. Everyone is safe. Where is Dad, Nicole and Mister P? wanted to know if everyone was as well as Philip looked. Shaken, white as a ghost but in one piece.

"The doctor is checking them out," the sister led me to the room where my husband was in bed. There did not seem to be too much wrong with him except a bruised and swollen face. He was not in danger. The doctor came there to find me when he was finished looking after Nicole and Wally.

"Your husband has a broken cheek bone which will need surgery. He will be taken to

Ruth Macklin

Mackay in a couple of days to have it fixed. Your daughter has severe facial wounds. It is badly bruised and rather swollen. I believe her jaw is also broken in more than one place but can't see too much at the moment. We are waiting for the ambulance to come back to transport her to Mackay."

"Can I see her?" I was taken to the room where the nurses were trying to make her comfortable and pain free.

When I walked into the room I could see no resemblance to the daughter I had seen a few hours before. Her face was broken, bruised and swollen to about twice its size. I would not have known it was her in the bed if the doctor had not been there with me. I could not believe she looked like that and Philip only had a blood nose. May be because Philip was on the back seat of the car and had held on to save himself when the car rolled. Nicole had been sitting in the front seat in the middle. Her face had been smashed into the dashboard and probably the windscreen.

I asked about Wally and was told he was being taken through to Mackay as the doctor thought he had a problem with his neck. The two men were hanging upside down when the truck driver found them. Both had to be let down out of the seatbelts.

"Has his wife been told?"

"I have rang her to let her know what has happened. That Wally will be sent through to Mackay."

"How long before they will have to go?"

Ruth Macklin

"Once I have them ready to travel they will go.'

"Fine. I'll go let the rest of my family know what has happened. Pick up Kath. Then

we will head straight through to the Base Hospital." I went back out to collect Philip who

had been sitting with a face washer over his nose to stop it bleeding. Went to my parents

home where I filled them in on what was happening, then left Philip with them and the

other three girls. Then I went to collect Kath before I headed for the hospital. I didn't

usually drive fast in normal times but this was not normal time. My foot went down on

the accelerator and I drove fast but with care, slowing when the signs said to slow. I didn't

want to be the cause of another accident in the same day. We arrived at the hospital

around the same time as the ambulance. We were walking into the emergency department

as the ambulance men were unloading the two patients. We had to sit and wait until we

were called to be told the new of their condition.

After all the x-rays had been taken and other tests done we were called in to be told

what was wrong. The doctors talked to Kath first because they had finished with Wally.

"I'm afraid you husband has a bone cracked in his neck. It will heal with careful

treatment. He will not be allowed to move his head for six weeks. We are going to put his

head in a brace to support his head,the doctor explained there were no other injuries.

"Will he be able to go home?"Kath wanted to know.

"No. We have to drill a hole at each temple to insert the rods to hold the cage in place

so the neck cannot be moved. He has to wear it for six weeks while laying flat on his back. He will not be able to move at all. He will be fed and given fluids." The doctor

explained how they were going to fit the frame and what it would look like. It would

look like a space helmet but not shut in.

Then came my turn to get told the bad news. The doctor told me there was not much

they could do that night except observe how Nicole went through the night.

"Nicole has a broken jaw which she will have to be sent to Brisbane to have wired

together. She may have other injuries as well we have not yet been able to find. That was

a nasty bump she has had to her face. We should know more when the swelling goes

down. She will be taken over to the children's ward soon."

"We'll stay until the both of them are settled into their rooms."

"We'll give you a call if either of them change for the worse during the night." Once

both patients were settled into their rooms we did our journey back home to wait for

news.

On Sunday afternoon I went back to Mackay to see how Nicole and Wally were.

Nicole was worse. She was twisting and shaking all parts of her body. She did not know I

was there by her bed. I could tell things were not going to plan. Nicole did not answer

when I spoke to her.

"Has something changed with my daughter?I asked the nurse. ?he was not doing all

that jumping last night when I left."

"The doctor has been to see her and has been asked to be kept informed of any changes. At the moment there has not been much change since last night."

"You will ring me if there are any changes? Does not matter what time it is."

"I'll let the doctors know you want to be called with any changes." I left the hospital and went out to the car where my mother had been waiting with some of the children.

"How is Nicole?my mother asked, as soon as I reached the car.

"Not too good." I shook my head from side to side to emphasise I was not too happy with her condition. "I think she is worse than she was last night. I don't think I will be getting too much sleep tonight. I have a feeling I will be called back to the hospital."

It was decided on the way home that the children should sleep at my parents home in case I was called out during the night to go to the hospital. Just as well because in the early hours of Monday morning, in the freezing cold, I received the phone call I had been expecting.

"The surgeon would like you to come into the hospital. How long before you can get here?"

"I will take about forty-five minutes. Sooner if there is not too much traffic on the road. Or fog."

"Come straight up to ICU. The surgeon will be waiting to talk to you. We are preparing Nicole ready for surgery."

I dressed in what warm clothes I could find, shoes, grabbed my purse and keys and headed for the hospital. There was not much traffic, and fog only hit in some places but

Ruth Macklin

not too thick. Took all the back streets with out traffic lights to make the journey quicker. Within twenty-five minutes I was racing through the deserted hospital trying to find my way up to the ICU ward. I knocked on the door still panting to catch my breath.

"I'm Nicole's Mother. I got a call to come to the hospital." I told the nurse who opened the door. I was led into the room where the nurses were preparing Nicole for surgery.

"I'll give the surgeon a ring to tell him you are here." The nurse went away to ring the doctor while I spoke to the other nurse.

The doctor was soon at the ICU ward to explain what he planned to do. Nicole has some bleeding in her head which is building up pressure. The pressure has to be relieved or it wall crush the brain. I am going to put a couple of burr holes into the base of the skull to release some of that pressure. There is a form for you to sign for permission to operate. I'll talk to you after the surgery. The doctor went off to be ready for when Nicole was wheeled into surgery.

Ruth Macklin

Chapter Fifteen

I stood beside the gurney on which Nicole was to be wheeled to the operating theatre when the nurse had finished preparing her. While the nurses worked I helped hold Nicole on the bed as her body kept jerking. The pressure on the brain from the blood build-up was causing her body to do this. Then it came to the last part to be done. Her lovely hair. It had to go. The nurses looked at me when the scissors were picked up ready to begin their work.

"Would you like to go out side for a moment?I looked puzzled at the nurses. ?e have to cut off all her hair and shave the scalp. We don? want you passing out."

"Thanks. But I'll be fine. You do what you have to do. Don't worry about me." I gave them a tired smile to let them know I would not faint on them. Or scream at them for what they had to do. The cutting and shaving of her hair had to be done to save her life. Hair would soon grow again. Would have been different if the doctors were going to cut off a leg, or arm. I stood there to hold Nicole still without hurting her injuries while the hair was hacked off with scissors. Clipped then shaved with a razor to make sure there were no bits of hair to get into the wounds. Then her head was washed. Not long after that Nicole was being rushed out of the door toward theatre.

One of the nurses showed me to the family room where I could make myself a hot

Ruth Macklin

drink, or have a sleep. I curled up on the sofa and went to sleep. Someone must have come to check on me because I had a blanket covering me when someone came to wake me after the surgery was finished and Nicole was back in ICU.

"The pressure has been released for the time being, I was told. But we don't know where the bleeding is coming from. We are not equipped here to find out the cause. We are making plans to have her flown to Brisbane on the first available plane. The doctors down there will find the bleed and also fix the broken jaw.

The sun was coming over the horizon when I walked out of the hospital to find my car to head home to tell everyone what had happened during the night. I was tired from lack of sleep and all the worry. I would not be able to travel with Nicole when she went on the plane because I had to organise a lot of things at home. Until it was time to go back to the hospital I had been packing and making sure the girls had all they needed while I was away. Philip I decided would be going with me. Didn't want to be worried about what he was up to while I was away.

I went back to the hospital to be with Nicole until she was taken to the airport. Was there when they put her on the plane. A couple of seats had to be removed on a normal flight to fit the bed in and all the machinery which had to go with her, and her escort. I went back home to catch up on some sleep until it was time for the children to come home from school. Transported the girls with their clothes over to my parents. Philip and I had something to eat and went to bed early.

Ruth Macklin

Philip did protest a bit about going to Brisbane because we had to drive past the place

where the accident happened. I knew that was his reason so I told him if he was asleep he

would not know we had gone passed the sight. To keep me awake I put a lot of cassettes

in the car so I would have music. There would be a lot of places I would not be able to get

radio reception.

We were up at midnight ready to leave while everyone else were still asleep. In places

we had to drive slow because of the thick fog. It was thick like pea soup by the time we

reached Miriam Vale. I had to stop for a while at the rest area until it thinned then set off

once again. It should have been a happy day because Nicole's birthday was that day.

Instead she was in a Brisbane hospital having operations on her eleventh birthday.

By mid afternoon we had arrived at the out skirts of Brisbane where we were going to

stay with relations. Joan had been in to be there when Nicole arrived on Monday. She had

to sign the papers for the operations as I was not there. The operations could not wait

until I arrived there. On the Monday afternoon one team of doctors operated on her head

to find the bleeding. The burr holes had kept the pressure down but they had to find the

cause. The side of her scalp had to be cut open so the doctors could stop the vein from

bleeding.

Early Tuesday morning Nicole was taken back to theatre to have her jaw fixed. The

jaw was broken in three places. Each break had to be wired together to hold them in place

and as close as possible to alignment. Top and bottom jaws were them wired together so

Ruth Macklin

she would not be able to move them. Nicole would have to live on liquid food until the

wires were removed and she could eat soft foods. She had not been long back in her bed

when we found our way to where she was in the children? ward. I stayed for a few more

days until the doctors told me she was out of trouble.

"Nicole will have to stay here for a few weeks until we are a hundred percent she is

well enough to travel. She should be right to go straight home when she leaves here. She

had been given a few knitted caps to wear on her head once the bandage and stitches were

removed. Hats she would wear to school through the winter months, or longer, until her

hair had started to grow."

Philip and I had the long drive back to Sarina. I was over tired and kind of lost when I

arrived home. I had been running on my strength and very little sleep for a whole week.

Everything seemed so unreal. My husband had had his cheek fixed and about to be sent

home from hospital. My strength tank was running on empty. I could of sat down and

cried but there was no time to do that as I had to catch up on work I had not been there to

do for the past week.

Just over three weeks later Nicole was released from Brisbane hospital and flown

home. Her face was back to near normal. At least she looked like Nicole. I had gone to

the school to explain about what had happened and how she would not have hair when s

he returned to school. The Principle and teachers had explained to all the children what

had happened to Nicole. That they were not to make fun of her with no hair because it

Ruth Macklin

was not her fault. So a lot of the student wore knitted caps to make her fit right in with the rest of the school.

In the years which followed Nicole had to have minor operations to have the wires removed to let teeth grow through. Wear braces on her teeth for about eighteen months. Then there were all the doctors and lawyers to see when it came time to set the insurance claim into action. Specialists to see to make sure of the facts of the claim. until finally the case was all over. When all the legal process was completed, monies were taken out for different treatments she had done, what money was left was put in a trust fund until she reached the age of eighteen. At that time the money was hers to do with as she pleased. The courts may have decided she should only get a certain amount for her suffering, pain and damaged done to her in the accident but they were not there to see what she looked like at the time of the accident.

On one of our flights back from Brisbane as the aeroplane flew above the thick, fluffy white clouds, Nicole asked,?an you walk on the clouds?"

"No. You would fall through to the ground. The aeroplane would not be able to fly through the clouds if they were solid."

"Oh. They look solid from way up here." Our home was a busy place. There were always people, or children, visiting or staying with us. Most times it felt as though we lived in a busy railway station, or an airport, with people coming and going at different times of the day. We had an open house. Not many people were turned away. Even

Ruth Macklin

though some of them I did not trust. They were friends of my husband. Fine when they were sober but not trust worthy when they were not. Because one young guy who had been allowed to stay at the house for a few day we had the police come to search the room he was using, for drugs. They didn't find any but it was the thought of once again I had the police coming into my home to search for something. I had nothing to hide so I let them search his luggage, and the room, he had been sleeping in. I made sure he left the house as soon as possible before he could cause any more trouble. With the police search, I had a good reason for telling him to leave my home. Didn't want him there to corrupt my daughters, or my son any more than he was at that moment.

Our life seemed to settle into a busy routine. Going to work. Helping with bingo and selling raffle tickets. Taking children where they needed to go. We were on a merry-go-round where we occasionally we touched base. I would have liked to live at a slower pace to be able to relax and do something for myself for a change. It seemed I was busy doing things for family and other people. I no longer had time to do one of my many interests which was writing. Had done a course to help but with family worries and stress, lack of time, I was not able to continue with writing. The stories I wanted to write were all wiped from my mind. The stories had been buried deep down where I could not retrieve them. So my writing was put on hold to be a busy wife, mother, and friend.

My life seemed as though it was in a deep, dark, rut where I could not climb out of because the walls were too deep, and getting deeper with every day. I was just a machine.

Ruth Macklin

Work! Work! Little sleep! Most of the time I lived on my nerves. From all this came an

ulcer and many other health problems. The doctor seemed to be finding all these different

problems. With each new tablet the problems grew because there were things in the

tablets which I could not have.

Near the beginning of November, 1985, Jody read an add about a guy starting up a

writing group in Mackay and wanted me to take her along to the first meeting. She was

thinking of joining. Said it would be good for me to get back into writing. We went along

to the meeting but after a couple of times Jody did not want to go. I joined. The group

was just what I needed. Different people to talk to about other things other than railway,

children, and what work was next on my list. I found the first few meeting stimulating.

The people were easy to talk with and discuss writing. We were friends who had an

interest in writing. Other topics were left behind when we walked into the room. I thought

now I had something to do for myself for a change.

My few weeks of happiness were shattered. On the first Sunday in December tragedy

struck. Robert did the ambulance raffles at the hotel. He had been drinking while he was

selling the tickets and after he was finished. In the late afternoon he came home to say he

was going fishing. He and a mate were going to take the fishing net down to the creek and

set it. Even though many rumours had be circulating around town there were crocodile

sounds coming from different parts of the creek. To set the net across the creek the men

had to swim. Robert had already been washed down the creek with the strong tidal flow

Ruth Macklin

to be sucked under the pipes of the causeway. He could have been drowned. That experience did not deter him from going back.

Michelle and Leanne went with their father and his mate to the creek to set the net and sit there for awhile to see if the fish hit the net. They came home just on dark to have dinner. Robert had to go back later to get the net out of the water. He took another mate with him to be there to help. The girls stayed home. I was not too happy about him going back down to the creek in the dark.

"Leave it until morning,I encouraged, but I was nagging. So he went.

As Robert went to go out the door he kissed me. It was there in that kiss. I didn't know what the it was but I felt it. The coldness of loss. A cold shiver ran down the entire length of my spine as the car drove out of the driveway. There was a dark cloud of misery. A feeling I was seeing Robert for the last time. I told myself not to be silly and closed the door.

I had been reading a book on ESP and the book explained how to ready your future with a pack of playing cards. Michelle and Leanne wanted me to try to read their future. The reading was slow as I had not much of an idea of what I was doing. For both of the girls there was the death card and water was involved. I did not know what these cards all meant as I was only practising. Reading the meanings of the cards as I turned them over. No matter how many times we shuffled and placed the cards the same meaning came out in the reading. So it seemed there was to be a death with water involved at some stage. By the time we had reached the end of the next reading I began to worry because I thought Robert had been gone too long.

Then the telephone rang. I rushed up to the lounge room from the kitchen to answer it. The caller was my father.

"Did Robert go fishing?"

"Yes. He set the net this afternoon and went back to get it out. He was to take a mate with him."

"The mate is here in Robert's car. I can't get much sense out of him. He said Robert went into the water and didn't come out."

That cold feeling was with me again. "I'll be right over." I dropped down the phone raced back to the kitchen to get the car keys. The girls and I got in the car to go to my parents house.

By the time we got there my father had his boat hooked up to the back of his car ready to go to the creek. I rushed up to the street to the home of one of the Search and Rescue members, who also worked with Robert, to tell him Robert had gone missing. He was going to notify the rest of the team. I raced back to where my father was waiting to go. I led the way to the creek in my car. My uncle was ready waiting by the side of the road to go with us to the creek as my father would need a hand to get the boat from the trailer. When I showed them to the creek I knew Robert was going to I went back to my aunt? home to ring the ambulance.

Ruth Macklin

I waited in the car for the ambulance to come then I took them down toward the creek. My father was on his way back home with the boat. I went to get out of the car but my father told me to stay put. Not to come any closer. The ambulance drove around me to park beside the boat. When I seen them get into the boat I knew what was wrong. I was told to go home that there was nothing I could do.

"Go home. The police will be at your house soon to talk to you." The ambulance man explained to me.

I went back to my parent? home to tell the rest of the family the news. My life had fallen apart. I had to hold myself together. Had to be there for my children, and family. They would need me. Everyone took the news hard. I had no time to think. Michelle I had to rush to the doctor to get something to calm her. She was upset because she had not wanted to go back down to the creek in the dark. Thought if she had been there she may have been able to save her father. If any of the children had been there I may have lost more than a husband to the creek. I may have lost some of my children as well.

How my father had been so quick at finding Robert had been because Robert had entered the water on the top side of the net. The net held him there. Stopped him from washing down the creek with the ebbing tide. If Robert had been on the other side of the

net we may never have found him. The crocodile may have found Robert before the searchers could find him.

Ruth Macklin

Chapter Sixteen

As the hour was late there were no patients ahead of me as I rushed into the doctor's

surgery to find some help for my daughter. We had just made it there in time as the doctor

was about to shut the door and go home. I explained what had happened and the doctor

gave me some medication to help Michelle to be able to settle and have some sleep. To

settle her so she would not keep crying all through the night. I rushed home because I

knew the police would soon be there to confirm what I already knew. Coming to tell me

was just part of their job.

"I know," I told them, and watched the relief on their faces that they would not have to

explain what had happened. "I had to show everyone to the area I knew my husband had

gone fishing. I suspected he had drowned when I was told by the ambulance men to go

home. Thanks for coming to tell me."

"There will have to be an autopsy to find the cause of your husband's death before he

is released to the family."

Once the death had been confirmed I had to ring relations to let them know what had

happened. To ask what I would be able to do. Whether Robert's family would like him to

be returned to Melbourne to be buried with his first wife. Or if I were free to make the

arrangements for the service to be held at Sarina. Robert and I had only been married for six years but had shared a house for a couple of years before. I felt I should ask the father

of Robert? first wife what the family thought should be done.

"You are his wife now. It is to be your decision what you would like to do. Make what

ever arrangements you think would be best for the family and let us know when, and

where, the service is to be held."

When I had finally let all the relations know the tragic news I fell into bed to try to get

some sleep because I knew I would have a tough week ahead of me. There would be trips

to Mackay to make funeral arrangements. The Father at the church to work out what time

he had available during the week. A couple of days after Robert? death was Jody's

birthday. A happy occasion over shadowed by a sad one. I also helped to make food for

the people who came to the service when I found time.

The small Catholic church was packed with family, friends and workmates, to say

their farewells. Family from far, and away, arrived to be at the service. To be there for us

in our time of need of support. Understanding of our sudden loss. To talk about old time.

Friendships formed over the years. After the service those who wanted to went to my

parent? home for a drink and some food. Then once everyone had gone on their way to

their homes it was time to settle back into widowed life with a family to raise. Philip was

allowed to come down from where he was at the detention centre in Townsville to attend

the funeral but had to go straight back after the funeral was over. He had an escort to

bring him and to be there with him, then escort him back to Townsville.

Ruth Macklin

There was no time for me to grieve. I had to fully take over the reign to make sure my family survived. Had the extra expense of a funeral. Robert's work mates took up a collection to tide us through until the railway did a payout and I had been in to sign up for a widow? pension. A death certificate had to be taken to a lot of places to have things changed. There were a lot of things which needed attention straight away. Besides I had to keep my family going. Help them through a tough time in the children? young life. Life had to go on one day at a time. The empty space had to be filled with family involvement. Or other projects in the community which Robert had been involved with.

As most of the people who helped with the selling of the Sunday raffles at the hotel did not know how the sale of the tickets were worked out I had to fill in, because I was the one who helped work out how many tickets should be sold per dollar to recoup the money for the prize plus make some money. I went to do the book work while the others sold the tickets. It was time away from my family but I gradually helped the men to understand about selling the tickets and what they had to do. The process was slow but I won out in the end.

On one occasion when I went to the ambulance centre to a meeting I had not been there long when the fire siren began winding up to call in all the volunteers to come in to fight a fire. "Nope it's not our house," we all said, as the wailing kept going. Then the phone at the ambulance station began to ring. Thinking it was for a call out the officer went to answer the telephone.

Ruth Macklin

"The fire is at your house, Ruth." I thought he was joking at first. "That was your next door neighbour calling to get you to go home."

I up off the chair and was soon out at the car ready to start the engine when Michelle arrived. She had run all the way from home to tell me what had happened. Michelle had not even stopped to put shoes on her feet to protect them from the stones. She was out of breath and shocked about the fire. I waited until she had climbed into the car before I took off in a hurry to reach home to see if there was still a home left.

The television which sat on the air cooler in the kitchen began to send out smoke where it had shorted out when Michelle had the television on while doing her homework. Due to her quick thinking the house was saved. She used something to reach over the freezer to switch off the power point so no more electricity would get to the television. Then she ran next door to get them to ring the fire brigade to come to put out the fire. The fire in the television was still smouldering and sending out clouds of smoke. The heat also melted the air-cooler. Lucky the house was not kept locked.

People were every where when I arrived home. The house full of acid type smoke. Walls through out the house were black from smoke. One good thing there was no structural damage. No walls were burnt. The whole house would have to be cleaned. Wall, curtains, clothes, blankets would all have to be washed before anyone would be able to sleep in the house. The children went to stay with my parents. I slept in the back of the car which was an eight seater van. The seats were folded down to make me a bed.

Ruth Macklin

Did not want to leave the house unattended in case someone came to remove things during the night. The house could not be locked because the window beside the television had been broken.

After every one had left and I tried to get things out of the house for the children to go to school, the smoke, and shock of the fire, made it hard for me to breathe and my chest got sore. I took myself off to the doctor to get something to help me get settled so I would be able to sleep, and get my breathing back under control.

Even after cleaning everything in the house the strong smell seemed to stay in the grains of the wood. I spent days cleaning as well as all the other things which I had to do. Besides I had to have the damage assessed before I could get rid of the damaged items and then I had to go shopping to have them replaced.

I finally become sick of being the bunny to do all the work and got out of all the other things over time. Kept helping with the bingo and the raffles. Then as the children became older I had more places to take them. Michelle went away to study in Townsville. I had to drive her up to Townsville with all her belongings she needed for her flat. She shared with a couple of other girls. Leanne and Nicole joined the navel cadets in Mackay which meant trips there of a Saturday for them to train. Their uniforms to have clean and ironed for each time. Take them in to Mackay to march on Anzac Day. Be at the base when there were march pasts to see which company had learnt the most. I seemed to be on the go all the time. The pace I kept seemed to go on forever. Sometimes I felt I was

Ruth Macklin

passing myself as I came in or out of the door. Like being in a revolving door. Go in one way and straight back out the door.

On one occasion when I went to collect them from their training Leanne and Nicole came rushing out to tell me their exciting news. We're going on a ship. Two days we are going to be away. We?l be able to run the ship with the sailors."

"Are you now? When is this suppose to take place? Who? all going with you?This seemed a bit risky to me. All those teenage girls going on a ship full of sailors. Not that I have anything against sailors. I just wanted my daughters to stay my daughters until they were ready to leave home to make a home of their own. Not that I didn't have trust in them. It was just the situation of putting impressionable young girls with a ship of guys who had been away from their families for some time. I didn't have the heart to tell them they were not allowed to go. I had to trust in them to do the right thing.

A couple of weeks later the Jarvis Bay docked in the harbour in Mackay on its way down the coast to Brisbane. All the boys, and girls, had to be in at the Mackay harbour early with all their luggage to last a couple of days. The parents were all there to see their children on to the ship and wave them good bye as the ship weighed anchor to leave the harbour on the full tide. Crossing our fingers we would see our children in a few days. Worried none of them would fall over board into the ocean. Not get hurt in carrying out

their duties on the ship. Most of the parents came from navy families and knew what to expect. I just had to pray everyone knew what they were doing and keep my daughters safe.

Ruth Macklin

All the children, or young future sailors, were given duties to work beside the sailors and do the work in the running of the ship day, and night, until they arrived in the port at Gladstone, where the children had to get off the ship to return home. Buses were waiting there for the ship to unload the children to return them to their destinations. Some were dropped off at their home towns as the bus made its way back to the Mackay port where their parents would be waiting to collects them. I waited at the bus stop for the bus to arrive. Both girls were excited about their trip but their were very tired.

"I got to steer the ship during the night watch." Leanne was so thrilled she had been given a chance to steer the ship. She was more excited about that then much else about the trip. "I didn't even let it go off course." So proud she could handle such a feat but tiredness won out once they had arrived home, showered ready to fall into bed to be up to go to school in the morning.

For days we were told of all the jobs the both girls got to do on the ship. The food they had been given. For awhile I thought I would have a couple of sailors but along the way life changed along with their minds of what the both of them would like to do. Nicole I though would make it but I think the main problem she didn't was because of the problems left behind from the accident. The burr holes and the broken jaw were the problem. Diving in the ocean is out because of the pressure under the water.

I was still busy helping with the raffles at the hotel. Every Sunday I had to collect the prizes to take to the hotel and get the tickets ready for selling when I arrived. I had a table

Ruth Macklin

in the lounge room. The men would walk around selling the tickets then bring the money

back to me to be counted once we had finished selling for the day. I had to have the next

lot of tickets ready to sell by the time the draw of the last tickets and the prizes given out.

One day I had a feeling of being watched as I worked. I finally looked up to see why I

had this feeling of being watched. There in the bar at one of the tables sat a guy with

some of his friends who watched me as I worked. He couldn't be looking at me, I thought.

I turned my head away from the table not giving him a sign I would be interested in him.

Not wanting to encourage him if he was interested. I had no room in my life for a guy.

My life was too full. Family came first, my writing which I had kept up since I joined the

writing group. I went to the writing group every Monday night. Had to fit in the writing

between work and family. It was the one night I had to myself to be with people who

wanted to do the same as me.

Everyone who attended the writing group brought a different level of writing skills.

Some wrote short stories and others like poetry. We were all given a say about each

other? work. Commented on how we thought the story could be improved, or whether it

should be left alone. Every comment was taken home for the writer to try to fix the

problems with their story. The more advanced of the group did editing of the work.

People came and they would also leave because the group was not what they wanted, or

left because they could not take some of the comments.

Fred! Fred could be the hardest of all. At one time he had been a reporter. He was also

Ruth Macklin

doing research for a book he had been trying to write. He had pages, and pages, of the story but he didn't seem to be getting to the finish. Work was not stopping him from getting his writing done. Bending the elbow I would say was the main reason he did not get too far. He could be too harsh on the people he should have been encouraging to continue with their writing. Fred would come at the writer of the story with both barrels blasting. He tore some of the stories to pieces, and the person? character as well, like a lion tearing in to its latest kill ripping the meat from the bones. There was no thought for the fragile or a new person trying to become a writer.

We all dreaded when it came time for Fred to make his comments on our work. One night he ripped my story to shreds and my character as well. You have a very big chip on your shoulder. You don't even like men,he blazed away at me. How he ever got such an idea from an innocent little story I don't know. All the members of the group looked on stunned by what he had to say. Most I think were waiting for me to get up to walk out crying, or flatten Fred with an almighty blow to his chin. No one would have blamed me if I had. I stayed put. I was not going to show such an arrogant person he had upset me.

If you had your work reviewed in early in the night Fred was not too bad but later he would get bold to say a lot more about each person? work. I always wondered why Fred changed during the night. Fred kept going out of the room which we all thought was a trip to the toilet. No. Fred did not go to the toilet. He may have visited on his way out to his car. I had to leave early one night when Fred had gone on one of his walks. He stood

Ruth Macklin

beside his car with the front passenger? side door open and in his hand was a bottle of rum. There was no mistaking the label on the bottle as the street light shone down on the bottle.

From that night on I watched how many times Fred took trips out of the room and watch the change come over him. I knew he would be going out to his car to have another sip of courage. How he never got pulled up by the police on his way home is a wonder. He would have been well over the limit. How he never caused an accident.

"Fred must have a weak bladder,"someone suggested, one night.

"He's not at the toilet. He will be out at his car, " I suggested, with a knowing smile on my lips. All eyes turned toward me. "Fred will be having a swig from his bottle of rum." When Fred did return members watched him closely and the people sitting next to him could smell the rum on his breath as he spoke. They knew I had been telling them the truth. Not long after the night Fred had been exposed his visits to the group were cut back and he finally stopped coming. At every meeting Fred did not attend there were great sighs of relief he had not turned up that night.

Ruth Macklin

Chapter Seventeen

I did get a little side tracked but I am now returning to the guy in the hotel. The guy

with the black hair, cheeky smile and the brown eyes with the golden flecks, devil's eyes,

which he used to entice females of all ages to let him take them to bed;or any place where

he could have sex with them. When Darrel had been drinking he didn't give a damn who,

or where, as long as he got his fix of sex. I didn't know he was like that when I first met

him but I soon learned Darrel used those come to bed with me eyes to his advantage to

win over the female to his way of thinking. Most of the time Darrel thought he was the

rooster of all but he didn't know all the females were the ones who were doing the

chasing without letting him know what they were doing. I don't think he was wise to all

the tricks the females pulled to get him for their own. Over the time I watched how they

operated to get rid of one another and curry favour from him.

Maybe the women thought Darrel would be good in bed, or they could say they had

been to bed with a guy who used to ride horses in rodeos for fun. Or the women could

have been not getting what they wanted from their husbands. Even wanted to spice up

their life with a change of bed partner. Possibly their husband could not give them

children. No matter what the reason Darrel was their property once they had hooked their claws into him. As he saw most days and nights through the bottom of a beer bottle, and the foggy haze brought about by drinking too much, he could not see clearly what had been happening around him.

In all the time I was acquainted with him I was his one true female friend who did not do things to impress him, or to catch him, because I knew he did not want to be caught. He also carried too much baggage. A wife who had left him for his best friend and taking his children away from him. Maybe that was a reason why he ploughed a wide field through the women in Sarina, from the legal age of consent to the married females. He didn't seem too fussy who he hurt in his endeavour to get what he wanted. There were many rumours circulating the town of women who claimed one or other of them believed him to be the father of their children, whether it was the truth or wishful thinking on their part to keep his attention for themselves.

In the beginning I liked the guy. After a short while I had stronger feelings, that is, until I realised what was happening. I did not want another husband who drank and to end up being abused once again, or to be wondering every minute of the day with which woman he had been while he was away from me. I stayed his friend, even looked after some of his children from time to time so he could get to see them, but I could not see myself living with a volatile person who could explode like a volcano in a matter of seconds. Whether it was with a look, said the wrong thing or touched him at the wrong time. One day in the crowded lounge at the hotel I came up from behind and touched him

Ruth Macklin

by accident, the next I knew I had a stinging cheek where he had hit me. From that day on my friendship with him went on a down hill slide.

Darrel may have wondered for a short while why I had started to distance myself from a loving friend to just a casual friend. The other reason was because there were too many back stabbing females who had their daggers pointed to my back because there were things I could do, or say to him, which they were not game to. They wanted him but they were also scared of what he would do to them if he had any idea what they were up to. Each in their own way schemed behind his back to get what they wanted. Me. I told how I saw things. Everyone wanted to be his friend until the crunch came and you could count his best friends on one hand. His true friends stuck by him to see him through the bad times.

Then came the car crash. He had to be taken to hospital with his injuries. Both of his hands in plaster for weeks as well as his body was very battered and bruised, his nose broken. For weeks he was laid up with all his injuries but not many there to help him except for his very close friends. There were not many females who wanted him then because he was of no use to them in his broken condition.

I stayed for the long haul. I was the one Darrel came to when he wanted advise about claiming for his insurance money for his accident. He took my advice. I went to the lawyer with him. Made sure he kept all his appointments and answered all his letters. The letters were sent to my address so I knew they would be answered. Rang him when I

Ruth Macklin

needed to make a time with him for appointments with the lawyer, or doctors. When I

told Darrel he had to be at a certain place at a certain time he knew he had to be available

if he wanted to collect his money for all the damages to his person in the accident. The

idea he would jump when I told him to was a sore point with all the back stabbing

females because they thought I was getting control over him and there would not be any

room for them. If they had only known there was no need for all the trouble. I was not the

threat to them having him. There was no room in my permanent life for a bed hopper.

One who didn't know who the last female was he had slept with. He had been too under

the influence of alcohol to remember their name.

Not once did I let it be known that I was being back stabbed by his female bed

partners, or their underhanded ways they used to undermine what each thought I had with

him. They were all jealous so they could not see what was there for them all to see. I

stayed right through the court case for him to see how much money he would be given

but I was not there to help him spend it when he finally had the money in his hand. All his

so called friends were there to help him celebrate. I kept away because my job of making

sure he did keep appointments were over. Free of the responsibility of seeing to

his need. Free to extract myself away from him. Free from any more trouble from the

back stabbers. Free to have my life back and to carry on as though we had not been very

close at one time.

He asked me to send in my bill for all the travel expenses and other items I had paid

Ruth Macklin

for while he was not able to do so himself. I did not add any extra for working under duress. The amount was itemised so there would not be any mistake of me being accused of helping, or being friends with him, just to get my hands on his money. Time was my own once again when I was not working. I quietly slipped out of his life all together but still spoke to him when I ran into him. I needed a break. Needed to make myself scarce to be able to think out what I should do.

So when Jody decided she was going to take an overseas holiday and wanted someone to go with her I thought it was a good idea. She was going to make all the arrangements. I was just going with for company. I had never been overseas in my life. Not once had I had a decent holiday where I could relax and not worry about work or family. So I found the money to pay for the trip. But in the end I was the only one who went on the holiday. I thoroughly enjoyed my holiday. The first holiday ever where I could go where I wanted to go and do what I wanted to do. Decide what I want to go to see. Not have to please everyone else. Not have to forget what I might want to do to be there for everyone else. It was time for me to spread my clipped wings.

The morning was wet and dreary the morning I woke to start the first day of my holiday. We arrived at the airport just in time for me to get my seat allocation and put my luggage through to be loaded on to the plane. Our departure was slightly late because of late arrival of luggage.

On the flight to Brisbane the journey was rough in places because of the air pockets.

Ruth Macklin

Long Hard Road

The plane was late arriving. I travelled on may modes of transport during the day such as a car, plane, taxi, bus and foot. It was quiet complicated and unreal at times as though all these things were happening to someone else; I was out of my element; moving in a strange world; different time; different dimension.

I had never been overseas to another country. I was about to head into unknown territory. As the weather would be freezing at the other end of the journey I packed, and packed. In the end I had a heavy suitcase and a small overnight bag. Lucky the suitcase had wheels.

Michelle met my flight when the plane landed in Brisbane. I went down to collect my luggage. That was a first mistake. I had labelled the big suitcase but did not have one on the over night bag as it was added last. Taking the one piece off the turntable I waited for the next one. Grabbed the one which I thought was mine and left. The luggage we took across to the overseas terminal and locked it in a storage locker to collect later. Then I spent the rest of the day with Michelle returning in time to put the luggage through customs.

On opening the overnight bag, which I had collected as being mine, found it did not belong to me. Mine had a winter coat and some other items but this one contained knickers, bras, and other clothing which in no way would have fit me. Michelle rushed the

bag back to the other terminal to find the missing one and have it back to me before I had

Ruth Macklin

to go behind the customs gate to wait to board the plane. I paced the terminal with worry. Could see myself missing the plane. Or part of my luggage would not make it. My mind kept telling me I should not have decided to go on the trip on my own. Should not be going to strange places where I didn't know anyone, didn't speak another language. I would surely get lost. Finally Michelle arrived back at the terminal with the right bag and some of the worry began to stop eating away my self esteem.

"I can do it. I can do it." I kept repeating over, and over in my head. I just had to keep repeating the same phrase each time I felt my confidence about the adventure begin to slip.

We were late getting on the plane because some cattle had to be loaded in to the plane. Some escaped being rounded up to be driven on to the plane. The cattle were running around the tarmac. If I remember correctly, there were twenty head of cattle loaded in the bottom of the plane. Not sure how far the cattle were to go. Our first stop was Singapore.

The flight was full to capacity with passengers, luggage, cattle and cargo. People returning to Singapore were loaded down with fruit and vegetables, presents. The plane finally ran down the runway to lift into the air. The only part of the plane trip I didn't like was when the plane lifted off the ground into the air and the coming back down to the ground. Once the plane level out I did not worry. I closed my eyes and went to sleep. The stewards had to wake me every time to eat, or drink.

When we left Brisbane the plane tracked its way across Australia, passing over Mt Isa, below Darwin then across the ocean to Singapore. Again we battled air pockets in several places during the flight. At times a ghostly mist blocked out view as it fogged the windows. The last of the rough weather came about two hundred miles from the Singapore airport. Dark ominous clouds passed below the plane as it shook. Glasses and food being quickly grabbed by their owners so they wouldn't spill on them, or the floor.

As we approached Changi airport, the lights of the town could be seen twinkling colourful shapes in the distance; the shapes became patterns of the layout of the city, it? streets and buildings. Changi airport was like a city with all the shops and plants through out the terminal; a city in an airport. There were buses there to collect the passengers to take them to their allotted hotels. The ride to the hotel was a wonder to see all the trees a light with fairy lights because Christmas was not far away.

Trees and gardens mingled with the concrete jungle. The street lights and trees combined did not look out of place. In the night the scene looked beautiful, not harsh; unnatural. The highway from the airport was like a tree with different branches until it became a jig-saw puzzle as we reached the inner city. The buildings loomed high in the sky. Most of the shops and hotels were decorated with the Spirit of Christmas. Everyone and everything seemed to move at a fast pace. The action seemed to go until the early hours of the morning and late starting the next day. Or maybe that was how it felt to me because I was used to getting up early each morning.

The shop owners try to sell you everything, and anything, bargaining with you to make

Ruth Macklin

more than one sale. The pollution from all the fast moving traffic makes breathing a

hard task when you are used to living in the country where there is plenty of fresh air. At

night Singapore was a tinsel town sparkling in all its glory but with the coming of the

morning sun the sparkle fades. The town is a mixture of country, nature and buildings all

fighting to live in the same place.

On the flight from Singapore we touched down at two countries as we tracked our way

to Amsterdam. The first stop was Bangkok. There was a passenger who wanted to get off

there so the Captain had to arrange for permission to land to let her off the plane. If

permission had not been forthcoming she would have had to carry on to another

destination then back track.

Our next stop was Istanbul. Snow flakes were falling as the plane came in to land. The

runway had to be cleared for the plane to land. We were not allowed to get off the plane

in either place. Not that I would have wanted to get off the plane at Istanbul because the

weather was freezing. It was warm in the plane until the door was opened to let the work

crew come in to clean and remove all rubbish. The cleaners were all rugged up from head

to toe when they came in to clean where the departing passengers were sitting.

The Turkish women were rugged up in thick woollen clothes, jackets, scarves over

their heads and tightly secured around their neck to keep out the cold and stop the wind

blowing the scarves off. High, leather boots were worn in which their slacks were tucked

to stop the cold going up the legs. We were there for a little over an hour. As we were

Ruth Macklin

ready to leave snow began to fall once again. It smashed against the plane as the plane

charged down the runway and lifted into the sky. I was very pleased when the doors of the

plane were closed because the cold could not come in side. You dress for cool when you

leave a hot country so are not properly prepared to stop over where it is freezing cold.

That was the first time I had ever seen snow.

We crossed many more countries before we reached Amsterdam. Some of the

countries we crossed were covered with snow. They were a winter wonderland. The view

was beautiful to see the peaks, ridges and valleys covered with snow, making the

landscape gleam white and clean as the sun shone down on the scene. Snow was still

falling but we were now above the snow but out side of the plane was about 60 degrees

below freezing so the television screen kept telling us. The ground covered in snow

looked magnificent from way up high. A winter wonderland which you see on some

Christmas cards. The scene sparkled from the sun shining on the snow not from the glitter

stuck to the Christmas cards.

Some of the passengers on the flight found out their video camera and were taking

pictures of the lovely view as the plane flew over. Lots of people moved from their seats

to look out a window. They must not have seen snow before either. There were a lot of

"Ohhh!" and "Ahhh!"coming from the passengers. I was lucky because I was in a seat

where I didn't have to move to look my fill of the beautiful scene. I am sorry I did not

have a cameras capable of taking pictures of the scene to bring back home to show my

Ruth Macklin

family some of what I had seen as the plane flew over.

Ruth Macklin

Chapter Eighteen

Most of the passengers were rugged up in their winter clothing by the time the plane landed at Schiphol airport, which is supposed to be classed as one of the best in the world. Those who had never been in a plane, which had landed there thought the pilot had come out of the thick mist and were about to land on the free-way. I didn't realise how wide the plane was until it came in to land. The runway was covered with ice and water, so the pilot had to put down the skis to help balance the plane as we skidded to a halt. The wings of the plane passed over the tops of the sheds built at the side of the tarmac. At a distance it looked as though the wing was going to hit the roof but it didn't.

My feet did not swell but I got a bit of a headache. My stomach gurgled from all the orange juice I drank during the flight because the flight attendants kept coming through with drinks and food to eat. During the flights we were given hot, steaming, cloths to wash our faces and hands. I slept most of the night hours of the trip, only waking when food or drink were handed out.

As I passed over my passport to the officer after leaving the plane, the guy said, "Kangaroo Island" cast him a nice smile realising Australia meant kangaroos to other people. Didn't want to say something which may have caused me not to get past his check point.

Ruth Macklin

The airport was massive and it looked as though they were extending it further with more shops, or places to stay, because of the construction site. Probably all in use by now because my holiday began in the middle of December 1991. You can travel from the airport by taxi, water taxi (boat), train or bus. I missed the bus because I had to find where I would be going to stay. One thing the travel agent who did my bookings did not mention hostels were not open in the winter months. Lucky I picked a nice taxi driver who took me to a reasonably priced hotel in the middle of Amsterdam.

I was taken to the Hotel Vondel which is situated in an excellent location in the quiet Vondelstraat. The hotel was in walking distance of all the places to see such as the museums and the most elegant shopping area. In the Vondel park and the exciting Leidseplein there are numerous restaurants, pavement cafes and fascinating night life. There is also special shuttle services to get you to all your excursions but I walked to all the places I wanted to reach to catch a bus to take me to the places out of the city.

I was very happy with the friendly service I received by all the members of staff as they were kind and helpful. They took good care of everyone who stayed there. Nothing seemed too hard. The hotel has about thirty rooms which all have private bathrooms, telephone and colour television. There are a lot of channels which cover many different languages. Breakfast was a tradition Dutch style which was included in the price of the room. There were boiled eggs, Salami sliced, toast, cheese, bread and tea or coffee. If asked they would cook meals or snacks but I never bothered them with requests such as

Ruth Macklin

different food. Coffee and tea were available most of the time so you just had to help
yourself.

The Hotel Vondel is a very old built building which has character and a feeling of
home. It is situated in a quiet small street away from the noise of the traffic. You can feel
the history in the building. The old fashion lifts which grind slowly to your floor. Or you
can take the winding stairs to your floor. Mostly I used the lift because it opened at the
room in which I was staying and didn't have to search out the room.

Once I had settle in to my room the first place I looked for was a shoe shop where I
could buy a pair of warm shoes to keep my feet warm and dry. A couple of pairs of gloves
to keep the hands warm. The scarf to put over my head and around my neck to stop the
chilly wind going down the neck of my coat. I went back to the room to dress warm then
went out again walking around to look at the shops. Stop at the street stalls to find a snack
if I didn't feel too hungry. Not once did I get lost and have to ask for directions on how to
find a place, or my way back to the hotel. I kept my eyes peeled for land marks which I
knew I would have to pass to get back to where I wanted to be.

On my way to the shops to buy what I needed a young guy on a bike stop me. Would
you like to buy a bike?I shook my head in the negative and kept walking. He was a bit
battered around the face so I had an idea the bike may have been stolen. Or maybe he had
other troubles and wanted money for drugs, food, or just wanted money to escape from
some family troubles.

Ruth Macklin

Coming back from the shops with the gusty wind blowing my hair, a tall female came walking up next to me, passed after awhile, stopped and turned around to look at me, then casually went on her way. Maybe she thought I was someone she knew. Or maybe the red colour of my hair was the interest. She may have been checking to see if it came out of a bottle.

So I would not end up with bad jet-lag I kept awake until night when it was time to go to bed as I was now in a different time zone. About two o?lock a slight mist began to cover the city and night clouds were making it dark. I didn't like to stay out in the dark on my first day there, didn't want to get lost. I went to bed and watched television but my eyes were soon closing once my body became warm as I snuggled under the blankets. The rooms were always warm because the heaters were let go day and night.

Even though I could not understand what most people were saying it was fun trying to piece together their conversations. There were some guys in the room next to mine. I did not see them in person. Must have been out on the town at some strip show. They arrive back at their room in the early hours of the morning stamping on the steps as they made

their way up to their room, instead of using the lift. By what I heard all of them were disappointed with the show because the woman did not bare her all. She did a strip in the show but walked away still wearing undies, or what ever covering she had not removed.

The next time I woke I thought the time was still early and was about to roll over to go back to sleep but decided to look at my watch. I got a shock to see it was eight in the

Ruth Macklin

morning and still very dark out side. The street lights were still on and with the darkness

the morning seem as though it was still night, something I got used to in a couple of days.

After breakfast I went wandering further afield walking around for about three hours.

When my legs became tired and didn't want to walk any more I went back to the hotel to

have a rest. It is easy to find your way around if you're observant and pick out land marks.

I was amazed when I came to my first canal. It didn't seem possible to have water

surrounding the buildings. Old and new buildings were cramped together. There were

market stalls on the footpath selling lots of different food to eat and other wears to buy.

The stalls seemed to be there every time I ventured out. Some of the buildings looked as

though they were built way back in the 16th century, maybe older.

On Saturday I went exploring in a different direction walking for hours looking at new

scenery. I came across a church with a gold crown on one of the spires which was called

Westerkerk. The building was very old but was in well kept condition and an eloquent

piece of architecture.

I found a McDonald's close to the hotel, a Burger King and a lot of little places to eat

and at a reasonable price for someone working to a budget, or only wanted to eat snacks.

Also good stop for a toilet break when you don? know where to find them in a strange

city. A good place to rest tired legs and to soak up the character of the country and its

visitors.

Sunday I went in a different direction and found some different shops. I was walking

Ruth Macklin

around window shopping. Not that anyone could see much of what the shops had because there were security grill pulled down over the display windows so thieves could not break the glass to help themselves to the mechanise. As I walked into the shelter section of the shop I heard what sounded like someone snoring. I turned to look to see where the sound came from to find some guy wrapped up in a blanket sound asleep. It looked as though he had come prepared to sleep out if he could not find a place to sleep. At least where he had selected to sleep was out of the chilly wind. Maybe he had one too many and didn't want to drive home.

Then I found where the canal tours started so I went for a trip in the closed in boat which lasted for an hour and a half. We travelled the canals and around the harbour. The trip was very enlightening. Cruised passed house boats on which people live and some had gardens which also floated. We did not get cold or wet while in the canal boats because of the roof and glassed sides.

In one part of the harbour there was a large sailing ship which has been turned into a museum for boating. The boat is centuries old and has been kept in good condition. The hostess on board the canal boat explained about the delights area of Amsterdam as we passed. There was a building which had been built in the shape of a boat but is privately owned so we could not go in to see the inside. At first it looked like a boat sitting on dry land. The smallest house in Amsterdam has one door and window in width but built four levels high. The hostess explained about the different gables on the top of the building

Ruth Macklin

neck; Italian and Dutch influence.

Some of the shops were open seven day of the week. Market stall line some of the streets selling food and wears. There was a flea market but it does not open on a Sunday. All the time I walked around the streets on my own not one person tried to beg, borrow, or steal from me. No one created a nuisance. May be because I was sensible by not carrying a large purse or bag. Never displayed I carried money on me. Most of my money and passport were strapped to my body in a cloth bag then tucked into my undies. I carried enough money for the day in a flat, small wallet which I kept in my coat pocket, then shoved my hand in the pocket as though I was keeping my hands warm. My camera I even carried in a plastic shopping bag which disguised what I really carried.

Not once did I feel threatened all the time I was on my holiday. I walked in places which I would never have done back in Australia. Don't know if I would still be able to do the same all these years later. I walked through misty, dark streets and did not feel any fear. Even on early mornings when I walked from my hotel through dark streets to catch a bus to go on a trip even when I walked past people coming out of night clubs around seven in the morning. There were never any hassles.

The next part of my journey was by train. I booked my seat to travel from Amsterdam on the fast express to take me through to Sweden. I walked to the train station as it was not too far. On my way back by a different street I found Rembrandt's museum and decided to go in and have a look at his art works. The walls were filled with paintings and

Ruth Macklin

sketches. Most of the painting looked real to life not blobs scrawled on a piece of canvas. You felt the people were able to walk out of the painting. You had to check in any overcoats or bags you carried, given a number to retrieve you items when you were ready to leave the building. I spent ages walking around looking at the paintings. The warmth of the building was also an incentive to stay awhile longer on a cold, misty rainy day.

From Rembrandt's Museum I walked through the arty area on my way where people had art works on display to sell to the public. I didn't buy any art because I had enough luggage with me. Little presents I could stick in with the clothes. Bigger pieces I would have had to carry. I returned to the hotel in the afternoon to sort out what clothes I would need to take with me to Sweden into a smaller bag and stored the larger suitcase at the hotel because I would be returning there to stay awhile longer, when I returned before my return trip home. Some may say I was stupid to leave most of my luggage behind at the hotel but I knew in my heart the owners would take good care of it for me. I felt the people were trustworthy.

The most puzzling and of some interest during the trip was the different ways the toilets and baths were operated. No body seems to mention these things before you leave for place you have never been. You should be warned what to expect or you could fall down a hole in the floor. To flush one toilet you had to stand on the button on the floor. Another one you had to straddle the hole while standing, or squatting. I backed out the door to find a normal toilet.

Ruth Macklin

Each canal in Amsterdam is said to be three metres deep but to the Dutch people the

tell the canals are one metre; mud one metre; bikes the next metre and the last metre is

water. Pigeon are everywhere. On one man? house boat he fed the pigeons and the birds

swarmed in from all directions. The pigeons were hanging on the man. His arms and back

were covered, legs and hat. A human bird perch as the birds squabbled to get their share

of the food. Another way of say it the man was dressed with birds.

From Amsterdam I went by train to Sweden which took all night. The train pulled out

about lunch time and we sped through towns, country side and countries. We crossed

through Germany and Belguim to get to Sweden. I was booked into a sleeper with about

four other people from Germany to Sweden. Had to change from one train to another in

Germany which was a rush. There was a railway worker there to grab us to get us to the

connecting train before it left without us. Trains leave on time. They don? wait for you. If

you are not on you just have to wait to catch the next one. There is a set time table which

is followed to the letter.

As the train crossed boarders to the next country we were all woken to produce our

passports to be stamped. I was lucky I carried my passport on my person so I didn't have

to get out of the warmth to search for it. If I ever get to do the trip again I would like to go

by bus and travel in the day time to get a better look at the country side. Or fly from

country to country then take bus trips to all the site of interest.

At some places along the way the train had to be loaded on to ferries to be transported

Ruth Macklin

to the other side of the water which was an experience. When we reached another section

of water we all had to get off the train to board the ferry to take us to the other side

because the wrong ferry had been sent to take the train to the other side. Had to get out of

a warm train to struggle with luggage through drizzling rain to get to the ferry. The trip

was short. On the other side we were hustled to get on to the next train which took us

through to Stockholm. Stockholm has a very large railway station with trains headed in

all different directions. There is a big waiting area where there are boards telling you

which trains go where and what time.

I found a cafe at the station where I bought something to eat for breakfast then waited

for the next train to take me to Upsala where my pen-friend lived. At least I did get to see

some of the towns and country the train passed through. From the station I went to see my

pen-friend and her family. She has a couple of cats. She had a young child who was cute

and friendly. I was taken to see a few different places before I returned to Amsterdam. I

would have loved to have more time and money to have stayed longer to see more of the

countries. I was lucky I had left when I did because there was a blizzard which killed a

few people.

The Stockholm railway station I remember well. I had returned from my stay in

Upsala where there were only a few hours of sun and the rest of the time the day was dark

so lights were on most of the day as well as the night. Building were heated to keep out

the cold. I was waiting for my train to take me back to Holland. There were a lot of

Ruth Macklin

people seated around waiting for their trains. There on one of the seats sat an elderly lady who was well dressed in fur coat and hat on her head. I had taken a seat on the opposite row of seats to her. Every thing was peaceful as people went about reading or talking to friends, or patiently waiting for their train to be announced as getting ready for boarding.

There were no people sitting next to the lady with the fur coat for her to talk to but some were close around in different rows of seats but not for long. People began to get up and move further away from her. No. She didn't smell. This lady began to raise her voice as she began to have a two sided argument with herself. She started off low but the further the argument with herself went her voice got louder. People rose as one. Picked up all their luggage and moved many rows of seats away from her. I stayed glued to my seat in wonder, amazement. I had never heard anyone have a loud two sided argument before. Not that I could understand what she was talking about. Maybe she was talking to an imaginary friend who she thought was deaf. The other people who moved must have understood what she was saying. I smiled at the reaction of the other people. No way they were going to get involved with the woman. My only thought was she did not catch the same train as I did. But alas, she caught the same train. We were in different carriages. I don? know where she got off the train as she didn't travel through to Holland.

I arrived back in Amsterdam just before Christmas where I went back to the hotel where I had left some of my luggage. I was given a different room but it was still comfortable and warm. The building had a life of its own. A history of which it could tell

Ruth Macklin

you if only the walls could speak. Some nights I felt as though the walls, or history, were trying to speak to me during my sleep.

New Year was a night I was pleased I did not venture out on to the streets on my own. Early the next morning I ventured out to have a quiet walk around the streets. Most time I walked to the square before I decided which way I would walk. The peaceful square looked as though it had not been peaceful during the midnight hour. Nearly every part of the square was littered with broken glass from bottles. Had to carefully make my way through the mess to get to the other side. I would not have liked to be the persons responsible for cleaning up the glass. The only advantage where the mess was it was all cobble and cement.

A few day later I left to return home. Had a long stop over in Singapore at the airport before our stop in Darwin. We arrived there in the early hours of the morning to drop off passengers. We seemed to be taking a long time to take off once again. An announcement finally came.

"Sorry everyone. But this is as far as we go at the moment. There is a problem with the plane. A part of the wing is missing and we have to wait for a part to arrive from Sydney."Moans could be heard echoing through the plane. "Those of you who have connecting flights please let us know so we can notify them of your late arrival. Please grab your hand luggage and head for the terminal. Once through customs you will be taken by bus into the city and booked into motels."

Ruth Macklin

We all grabbed our things to file out of the plane still half asleep. After all our luggage had been searched we were taken to our motels. Once my luggage arrived at the room the first place I headed was the shower. It had seemed like days since I had been to a place where I could have a shower. Next came breakfast before a short sleep. I went for a walk

in the afternoon. Just around the block, I thought. Didn't think I would make it back to the motel because the block seemed to go on forever.

Finally we were taken back to the plane fourteen hours later to continue on to the next leg of the journey to Brisbane. I then had to spend the night there because my plane had left hours before we arrived. The next morning I was on the first available plane to Mackay. Sad my holiday had passed so quickly but please to be home.

Ruth Macklin

Chapter Nineteen

To go to the next part of my story I have to regress to before I went for my holiday. My

family were at the age where they were leaving home one by one. I felt I needed to make

a few changes in my busy life so I decided to sell the house in Sarina to move out into the

country. My idea was to buy a couple of horses and a few animals. I found a place, which

needed a fair bit of work to straighten it to the way I had envisaged. Believed I would

have some time to myself to do things my way. Would be able to do work at my leisure

but I was mistaken.

I would go to work looking after a couple of children and doing work in the home.

While I was away from the house animals would start to appear. I started with two horses

I had bought just before I moved. Pigs appeared when my father and a friend returned

from a holiday, followed by chickens, ducks, geese and a cat which became jealous when

another cat came to the house and he ran away. The new cat was a female which soon

added to the collection of animals. The hens also began to multiply by bringing home

chickens from where they had hidden a nest in the scrub. Even the pigs were in on the act

having large litters of piglets. One sow produced thirteen piglets. One of the horses

produced a foal in the early hours one morning.

My place of peace in the country soon became a place of hard work and stress. I had to feed the animals and wash the pig pens before I went to work. Work all day and return home to feeding all the animals, cook and do other work. It seemed as though I had once again climbed on a merry-go-round.

As well as all the animals producing young so was Leanne. She began complaining she was taking so long to deliver her baby. She grew bigger by the day.

"Go down to the paddock," I would tell Leanne. "All the animals will show you how to deliver. They are all beating you and you had a head start. Even the sister-in-law had joined the race. All the animals had their babies before the girls did."

Leanne had a false labour and had to come home from the hospital. Brad had driven her to the ambulance station to get them to take her to the hospital because he didn't want to have to deliver the baby along the road between Sarina and Mackay. A few night later the pains started once again in the early hours. Leanne and Brad were walking around the house discussing who should take her to the hospital. Brad wanted the ambulance. Leanne wanted me to drive her to the hospital.

"Mum will get me there quicker," Leanne protested. "Look how much time was wasted last time while we had to fill out all the papers. Mum will have me at the hospital before the ambulance leaves the station."

"You won't get there in time if your mother drives. She drives too slow."

"Mum will get me there in time," I heard the loud whispered conversation as Leanne walked toward my bedroom door.

Ruth Macklin

"What's up?" I asked as her head came around the edge of the door.

"Having bad contractions. Will you drive me to the hospital? Brad wants me to go in the ambulance. They take too long."

"What time is it?"

"Four o'clock. Why?"

"I have to be back to take Nicole to work. I'll get dressed." I crawled out of bed to throw on some clothes to take the forty-four kilometre drive to the hospital.

Brad just shook his head when Leanne got in to my car. He went in their car. The first few kilometres I had to drive with hurried caution because the road was unsealed with loose gravel. Once I hit the highway I put my foot down. Slowed to pass through Sarina then took off toward Mackay. The forty-four kilometre drive which usually took over half an hour was completed within twenty minutes. I took all the back streets in Mackay where I knew there would not be traffic light to halt our progress.

"Wow! I didn't know your mother could drive like that,said Brad, as we made our way into the maternity section of the hospital.

"Told you so. I trusted mum to get me here on time." I waited around the hospital to nearly six before I had to leave to drive home, at a more moderate speed, to wake Nicole to go to work. She was still asleep when I arrived home to knock on her door to tell her it was time to get out of bed.

Ruth Macklin

"Your dressed early. What have you been doing?" came a sleepy voice, as Nicole made her way out from where she had been burrowed under the covers.

"What do you mean what have I been doing? You mean you slept through all the noise?" I rolled my eyes skyward as I shook my head. How could she have slept through the pacing Leanne had done.

"Where's Leanne? She's not in the lounge room," said Nicole as she sat down at the table for breakfast.

"You mean you did not hear the car go out of the shed?" The car in the shed was right next Nicole's bedroom window. It is a wonder the slamming doors of the cars and the starting of the engines didn't wake her. "I took Leanne to the hospital in the early hours. I have just returned home."

"Again. Has she had her baby yet?"

"She will probably be home again this after noon." I took Nicole off to work then came back home to feed the animals and do some work. When I had finished I thought I would go to bed to catch up on some missed sleep. Not so lucky. I hadn't long dozed off to sleep when the phone rang. I crossed my fingers as I went to answer the phone hoping I was not to be called into work.

"Hello."

"This is the sister from the hospital. Could you come in your daughter would like to see you."

Ruth Macklin

"It will take me about half an hour to get there."

"Not to worry. She won't be going any where." Within a short time I was headed back to Mackay to the hospital. I was bone weary. A couple of hours sleep would have done me the world of good. When mother's are needed sleep goes out of the window.

When I arrived at the desk to tell them who I was and who I had come to see I had a nurse saying. "Oh your the missing mum. Come through this way." I followed down a hallway to where I expected to be taken to a room to find Leanne in a bed. I could hear noises behind a door and thought someone was delivering their baby. The nurse opened the door to usher me in and closed the door behind me. There on the labour bed was Leanne a doctor sitting at the end of the bed and Brad standing to the side trying to keep cool. I didn't expect to be whisked into the labour room.

"Now we might see some action," chuckled the doctor. "She had to hold on until her mum arrived."

A wet face cloth was shoved in my hand to bathe the fevered brow while Brad had his hand squeezed as Leanne complained about the pain. Wanting the baby to be born so the pain would stop. I couldn't believe I had been allowed to go in to the room.

"Can't we hurry this up?" Complained Leanne, between contractions.

"You're the one in charge," said the doctor. "We're waiting for you to deliver."

Diversion. That was what was needed before Leanne could get over excited. I don? know what the doctor thought of the diversion but I had a captive audience. I went on to

Ruth Macklin

explain she should know what she had to do. The chicken and ducks had beaten her. The

pigs had delivered their litters. I told her she was the luck one as she would be delivering

one baby. Look at what the sow had to go through as she had delivered thirteen babies in

one go. The cat had had her kittens. She had to hurry if she wanted to get in the line

before his sister-in-law came to deliver her baby. The wild stories about where the

animals had to have their babies was a lot worse than being in the labour room. All she

had to do was follow the animals and deliver her baby. Leanne had calmed enough to

concentrate on what she had to do and in no time at all my grandson was born. Once

Mitchell had been born he was placed in my arms wrapped in a blanket until all the fuss

was over and the mess cleaned away. I stayed until Leanne was taken back to her room

then it was time for me to return to Sarina to spread the news and collect Nicole from

work.

   After the animals had been fed we had to return to Mackay for Nicole to visit her new

nephew before we were to attend the birthday party dinner for the Mackay writers.

Something told me to look down at the fuel gauge as we were coming into Mackay. I

nearly had a fit. The needle sat on the empty mark. Lucky for me I had a choice of a

couple of petrol stations before we would have had to walk. I had been on my third trip

into town in the one day. In the rush I had forgotten to keep a check of the fuel. I gave a

big sigh of relief as I drove into the driveway and turned off the engine. I don't know how

far the car had been running on the fumes in the tank. Best I didn't know. I fell into bed

just after midnight and was asleep when my head hit the pillow.

Ruth Macklin

With each day of my life which past I seemed to have less sleep and work longer hours. So when Jody suggested the holiday I soon agreed I needed to have a complete rest to be able to have a good think while I was away to sort out my life. To get rid of some of the work which had been keeping me busy. The more I tried to work the sicker I became. I needed to make some down time for myself.

I was still trying to think about how I should make changes when tragedy struck my life once again. I had just returned to the house from feeding the animals on the first Sunday in July. The wind had been whistling down the hill to the flat while I had been working. The wind trying to rip off my coat. My heavy rubber boots making it harder to walk against the wind. My hands were red and cold from putting out water for the animals. I struggled up the hill to the house thinking I would have time for a rest before having to cook a meal. Nicole would not be home for a couple of hours.

Not long after I had laid on the bed for my rest the phone began to ring. I cursed as I made my way to the lounge room thinking the caller would be someone wanting me to do something for them. The caller was my father. He was very upset.

"You had better get in here quick. Something is wrong with Jody. She collapsed on the floor in the shed screaming. Now she won't talk. Won't tell me what is wrong with her."

"I'll leave right now." I dropped the phone, grabbed what I would need to take with me then raced out to the car.

Jody lived with my parents in Sarina to be there with them in case they got sick and because she had a part time job. I had been talking to Jody on Friday and there didn't

Ruth Macklin

seem to be a problem with her health. If any one was to be sick I thought it would be my father because he was prone to having mini strokes. Or my mother who became very sick very quickly with blood poisoning. But I would not have expected to receive a call telling me Jody was sick. I made the trip in a hurry keeping a look out for a flashing blue light to come up behind me as I sped to my destination. I would have had a valid excuse if I had been pulled over for speeding. My daughter was sick and needed my help.

I pulled the car into the driveway, switched off the engine before opening the car door to race into the shed. My father paced around the shed keeping an eye on Jody to make sure she did not wander from there before I arrived. The moment I set eyes oh Jody I knew she was in big trouble. The light was on but no one was answering the door. Her eyes stared into space and she would not talk.

"Jody has had a headache all day. Nicole was to pick up some tablets at the chemist in Mackay and bring them when she came home. Your mother is in Mackay at bingo. I didn't know what to do." My father was in a big panic. I hoped this would not cause him to have another stroke.

I walked over to where Jody stood."Jody." She recognised my voice and her name. "Come on. I'll take you to the doctor."

Placing my arm around her shoulder I led her to the car and we helped her to climbed in to the front set then put on her seatbelt.

"I take her up to the doctor to see what is wrong. If he is closed I'll rush her straight

Ruth Macklin

through to the Base hospital."

The doctor's surgery was close and so was the ambulance centre so I headed the car
toward Mackay. I drove fast but careful. I kept talking to Jody as I drove but didn't receive
any answer. She sat there as though she didn't know what was happening, just staring
ahead at the road.

Once again I zoomed around all the back streets where there were no traffic lights to
get to the hospital as fast a I could before Jody had another turn and tried to escape from
the car while I was driving. Luck was with me and there was not too much traffic on the
road for a Sunday night. I turned into the parking area at the river side of the hospital and
parked as close to the door as I could. Knew not to park in a parking area because I knew
I would be a long time at the hospital.

Opening the passenger door to help Jody out she stood beside the car in a daze as I
locked the car before leading her through a door of the hospital to make our way slowly to
the emergency department. Jody followed where I led without comment. I found our way
to the nursing station and told her what had happened. She took us to a room before she
went to find a doctor. We were both seated on chairs waiting when the next stage of the
illness took over Jody's body. Her body convulsed as a fit took hold. I reached out with
my arms to try to hold her on the chair.

"Nurse! Nurse!" I yelled, in the hope someone was close enough to come to our aid.

A nurse and a doctor came rushing into the room as I struggled to hold Jody. Between

Ruth Macklin

the three of us we lowered her to the floor until the convulsing had stopped. From there

on it was panic stations. Help had to be summoned to help Jody from the floor on to a

gurney to be taken into the examination room where she could be checked out to find

what had caused the problem. Blood tests were taken. Even a spinal tap had been done.

Even though Jody was out of this world she still screamed as the doctor done the spinal

tap. They tried every test they could think to do. Before long Jody was rushed up to the

ICU ward where the doctors hooked her up to all these machines, drip lines put in,

catheter put in to collect urine samples and connected to the breathing machine which did

her breathing for her.

Nicole brought my parents to the hospital late that night to find Jody all wired up to

the machines. The shock of seeing a once healthy, happy person now depending on

machines to keep her alive. No matter how much we talked to her there was no response

except a twitch of an eyelid to let us know Jody recognised a voice but the eyes never

opened. I stayed after Nicole had taken my parents home until the nurses told me to go

home as there was nothing more which could be done until the morning when all the

specialists came to work.

As I made my way through the empty section of the hospital to find my way to the car

I became aware how cold the weather would be once I opened the door to the outside

world. Ghostly wisps of fog come with the wind from the river with a heavy dew

covering the car and the grass. I pulled my jumper closer to my body to try to keep out

Ruth Macklin

the cold as I made my way to the car. Climbing in side the car I started the engine to

warm the car and clear the windows before I moved out.

The trip through the town streets were not too bad at midnight with the thin wisps of

fog floating by in patches. Once the street lighting was left behind the fog became thicker.

Some sections were not too bad but in other areas I had to slow to a crawl because the fog

thickened making a white out effect of the surrounding area with only a few feet of road

to be seen. Even with the lights on high beam the ghostly swirls of fog locked out any

view except for the few feet of bitumen in front of the car. Tied eyes strained into the fog

to make sure I did not head off the road. Luck for me I knew every bend, bridge and rise

along the road between Mackay and Sarina. The times the car had travelled that section of

the road the car could have found its own way home.

As the sun rose to bring in a new day I dragged my weary body from my warm bed to

go to feed the animals before I would be able to return to the hospital. I packed some

clothes for Jody to take into the hospital in the hope she would wear them when she got

better. I had this feeling but there was always hope but some times wishing, hoping and

praying are not enough to get the loved one through to a healthy happier life.

I spent the morning beside Jody when the doctors or nurses were not attending to her

or doing tests. Family came and went during the day to visit Jody to see if there had been

any changes but there were none. Jody was slowly slipping away from her family. A CT

scan had been done but nothing showed on the x-rays of what had to be causing the build

Ruth Macklin

up of fluid around her brain. No medication helped to slow down the process. During the day and many long discussions by phone the powers-that-be decided to send Jody to Rockhampton by air ambulance to see a specialist and to have a special type of CT scan done with a special dye. The normal dye which many people have could not be used on Jody because the last time she had an x-ray with the normal dye she had formed blood clots. Any one allergic to seafood can not be given the dye. Jody could eat seafood but could not have some of the products used in the dye.

The arrangements had been made for the air ambulance to come on Monday night. I went home in the late afternoon to get some clothes for myself and organise with my father to feed the animals while I'll be away. Also told them I would leave the car at the hospital and the keys for someone to come in to collect it the next day. I went back to the hospital to wait for the transfer of Jody and myself to Rockhampton.

Jody had to changed from most of the hospital machines to the ambulance one to be taken to the airport. Things didn't look good when we walked out of the hospital to get into the ambulance. The cold weather had brought in a fog. The fog swirled around the side of the ambulance coating our clothes in the fine wet mist. Never in my life had I seen such a thick fog in a town. It was a complete white out. The flashing lights of the ambulance cast creepy dancing colour in the fog. The fog lights helped to keep us on the road as we travelled at a slow ten kilometres an hour to make our way through the streets to the airport. We finally made our way through the gate on the side of the airport where

Long Hard Road

the planes used to land before the new airport building was built.

We waited there listening for the aeroplane to circle the airfield and come in to land. The sound of the engine could be heard off in the distance before it circled but did not land. The pilot was refused permission to land because the fog had become much thicker making it unsafe for the aeroplane to attempt a landing. There was no way the pilot could find the runway even with the lights to guide him. He would have been flying blind until he had reached the ground. The mission was aborted and the pilot returned to Rockhampton. We had to make the slow trip back to the hospital to make another attempt in the morning.

The next morning we made the trip back to the airport to wait for the aeroplane to arrive. Shone shone brightly with no sign of the fog we had encountered the night before. A shock was in store for me when the aeroplane finally landed and rolled to a stop near the ambulance. How were they ever going to get Jody into the aeroplane. It was a toy. The ambulance seemed bigger than the aeroplane. There were all ready two people in the toy and Jody had to be placed in there with all her equipment. There would be no room in the toy for me to go with. The side of the aeroplane was opened and Jody placed in the tail section, quickly hooked up to machines before being closed. Moments later the toy coasted out on to the runway and lifted into the sky. I had everything crossed in the hope the aeroplane would be able to lift into the sky with the heavy load.

Arrangement had been made from the ambulance to the hospital for me to catch a regular flight. A ticket waited for me at the counter when the ambulance dropped me at

the new terminal. I had to wait for the flight to arrive which would take me to

Rockhampton. The aeroplane I was on landed over an hour behind the air ambulance. I

caught a taxi to take me to the Rockhampton Base Hospital. I went to the main entrance

to find out information where I could locate Jody. I explained how she had arrived and I

was her mother. The lady I spoke to gave me directions of where she was told I could find

Jody.

Setting off I wended my way through the hospital to find the section. I asked at the

nurse? station and was shown to the room which was not far from the nurse? station. The

nurse stood there telling me what had been organised since Jody had arrived. Test had

been set up to be done as soon as the x-ray was free. All hell broke loose. Jody had a

strange breathing sound as I stood by the bed then she began fitting. The nurse hit the

panic button bringing doctors and nursing staff rushing into the room. I was hurried from

the room to make room for all the emergency people.

Standing out side the room I heard what the doctors were doing to try to save her life.

The electric shock which made her heart begin to pump to live once again. Then a nurse

had been sent to take me to the family room away from hearing what had to do. Once

Jody had been stabilised she was rushed from the room to have her very important CT

scan to see what had caused the build up of fluid around the brain.

"Jody had been taken for her scan,the nurse told me. ☐ he will not come back to this

Ruth Macklin

section of the hospital. The doctor said she would be going up to ICU. Why don't you go

over to the Red Cross rooms across the road to book in to a room, have something to eat

and by then Jody should be up in ICU."

I went and booked in and had a quick shower to try to revive me from the lack of sleep

over the past couple of nights. Grabbed a quick snack at the shop on my way back to the

hospital to find my way to the floor where the ICU rooms were. I sat on a chair in the

corridor waiting for someone to come find me when Jody had been settled.

"You can come in now,said the nurse. He lead me past all the other beds where there

were very sick patients to the part where my daughter seemed to have more machines

hooked up to her than there had been in Mackay. I was given a chair to sit beside the bed.

"You can talk to your daughter as she may can recognise your voice. Hold her hand to

let her know you are there with her."

I touched her hand and I knew. Knew what I had not yet been told about the tests. The

space blanket which covered her also gave me a sign of what the answer would be. Jody

had held on to her precious life as long as she could until I arrived at the hospital before

she took the next turn around the corner.

At about ten o'clock the nurse advised me to go to have some sleep as there was not

much else could be done until the doctor had seen the tests results. ?e will give you a call

if there is a change in her condition during the night. So I was convinced to leave to get

some rest with the promise from the nurse I would be called.

Ruth Macklin

The cold winter wind whistled around me as I made my way from the Red Cross room to let myself in to go to bed. I was so cold I only slipped off my shoes before I crawled beneath the blanket to try to get warm. Didn't take off my clothes to put on a nightdress as I would only have to dress into cold clothes if I had to go back to the hospital.

During my restless sleep Jody came to me to say good bye. I felt her presence in the room as she came to tell me she would not be going home. She would be going to a different home where there would be no pain. Not to worry she would be fine. I must have then dropped in to a very deep sleep. The next I knew someone was banging on the door trying to wake me.

"Yes," I mumbled, as I forced my eyes to open and my foggy brain to work.

"There is a call from the hospital for you," said the voice from the other side of the door.

I scrambled from beneath the pile of blankets rushed to open the door, opened it to rush to the phone. In my haste to leave the room I forgot about locks. When I had finished speaking to the nurse at the hospital I went back to the room to find my shoes but could not get into the room. "Ohh! No," I complained as I turned the knob of the door. I went back out to the lounge room to find the person who had called me. "I'm locked out. The door closed as I came out. How do I get a key to get in?"

The woman went to find the manager to tell him what had happened so he came to open the door for me. "Thank you. I didn't think about the lock in my haste to get to the

Ruth Macklin

phone. I have to go over to the hospital." Quickly finding my shoes I grabbed the key to

the room and made my way over to the hospital.

Once I arrived at the ICU room I picked up the phone out side the room to let them

know I had arrived. The door was unlatched for me to open the door to walk into the

room and make my way to where my daughter lay on the bed, the noise of the breathing

machine sounding loud in the room. My eyes flicked over what I could see of Jody with

all the machinery, wires and tubes.

"Your daughter has had another fitting turn. The doctor has been in to see her. He has

made arrangements to do some more tests, and an x-ray in the morning. He would like to

talk to you when the tests have been completed."

"Will they know what is wrong with her? Will they be able to operate to release the

pressure?"

"I really can not say. The doctor didn't tell me what he intended doing. You can stay

for a short while but then you will have to leave as I have to do obs and a few other things

the doctor ordered."

I reached out to hold my daughter? hand but it was cold. Not cold weather cold but a

different kind of cold. Jody's body lay there hooked up to the machines which were

keeping her organs working but her life and soul had left. I left the room a short time later

with the firm belief the new in a few hours time would not be good. Didn't get much sleep

when I returned to the room and was up early to have a snack before I returned to the

Ruth Macklin

hospital. I didn't pick up the phone to let them know I was waiting because I knew there were special tests which had to be completed. I didn't want to interrupt what had to be done.

Finally, the doctor and the sister came out to tell me what had been found. I could see by the looks on their faces they were going to confirm what I all ready suspected. I stared at them in shock but holding myself together on a tight rein so I would not crumple and fall to pieces. I had to look after my daughter.

"We have completed the tests on your daughter. The results were not good. The fluid which kept flooding into her head has squashed her brain. The machines are doing all the breathing for her. If we were to turn off the machine her body will shut down. Your daughter is what we call Brain Dead. The brain is no longer working. Do you understand what we are telling you?asked the doctor, not sure if I knew what he had been explaining to me because I had been nodding and staring as he talked.

"Yes. My daughter is dead. What happens now?" The both of them looked at me waiting for me to start screaming, or accusing, because Jody would not be going home a healthy, happy person.

"The machines can be turned off. But before we do that we would like to know if you, or your daughter, have ever spoken of organ donation? You could help a few people with the donation of her organs which are still healthy."

"No it was not discussed but I do know she had the box ticked on her licence."

Ruth Macklin

"Would you consider agreeing to them being donated? We would have to make plans for the transplant team in Brisbane to come up here to do the retrieval and find the suitable people to receive them. The machines would stay on until the team arrived to keep the organs working."

"Fine. Do what you have to do." The doctor left to organise what had to be done. The sister stayed with me to explain what arrangement I would have to make toward a funeral. Papers to sign to say I had agreed to the harvest of the organs to be given to patients to save their lives. The team would not arrive until later Wednesday night so they would not upset other operations planned for the day. A chance to get the patients prepared in hospital.

As I waited for the lady to fix all the paper work and ring the funeral home to have Jody shipped back to Mackay my cousin Rhonda came to the hospital to find out how Jody was as she had just found out I was at the hospital.

"How's Jody? Has she improved?" I shook my head in the negative. "What are the doctors going to do?"

"Nothing they can do. The doctor has been out to see me. Jody has been declared Brain Dead."

"Ohh, shit!" Rhonda throw her arms around me and the whole story poured out as the first of my tears began to flow.

"Have you rang home to tell your mother what has happened?"

Ruth Macklin

"I have just finished signing all the papers. I have given permission for Jody to donate her organs. I dread having to ring to tell my mother the bad news" .I stood to slowly walk down the corridor to where I knew there was a pay phone. My weak legs just holding me up. I felt as though I had aged many hears since Sunday. I aged with every tragedy. I had a feeling I would be well past my used by date before my age caught up with me.

"How's Jody?"was the first words my mother asked.

"Not good news I? afraid. Jody won't be coming home." The words had no sooner left my mouth when I heard my mother scream. When I could I explained what I had been told. Next I was being told my parents were coming down from Sarina to Rockhampton. A friend had offered to drive them down to see Jody to make sure I had been telling them the truth because they could not believe she had died.

Rhonda and I were taken in to see Jody where a small ceremony was held by her bedside. It was all done with gracefulness and in thought for the family who were there. Some of the nursing staff stood there as well. Jody looked peaceful as though she had just gone to sleep.

My parents arrived a few hours later at the hospital and I took them up to see Jody. I had told the nursing staff we would be all in to say good-bye to Jody before we left to return home. The nurse told us we could stay until the time came to turn off the machine before going into theatre but I knew the strain would have been too much for my parents to take. The shock of hearing Jody had gone was enough for one day. I didn't want to have my father having another stroke while watching the machine being turned off. We

Ruth Macklin

went home for me to organise things while waiting for Jody to be returned home. An autopsy had to be done to find out what had caused the fluid to keep building. None of the scans had found the problem. The doctor found a tumour hidden at the back of the brain where the scans were unable to pick it up. Once Jody had the first attack there was no way to help her to live.

On the thirteenth of July Jody was laid to rest. The same date as her brother had come into the world but never got to see it. Jody lived a short twenty- two years and a few months. She never made it to her twenty-third birthday.

Ruth Macklin

Chapter Twenty

Donations. There are different types of donations. A few were not happy because I agreed to the donation of Jody's organs. They seemed to think of donating organs as macabre. To me this was the last thing I could do for Jody. To carry out her wishes to be an organ donor. No one said too much to me but the looks told the whole story. I looked at the donation as not completely loosing my daughter. There would be more of Jody in Australia but with a different name. While those people were still alive from the donation Jody would like on.

Jody was the one happy with what I had done. I have been told by a few of the believer people that Jody told them she was pleased I had carried out her wishes. Since then I have accepted what I did was the right thing to do. I had to deal with my loss but the donations helped others to live a more normal life than would have been possible if they had not had their transplants. People from Rockhampton to Melbourne received some part of Jody.

A book I read recently was a story about donor families receiving letters to thank them for the giving of the gift of life to their loved ones which is done through the transplant team. Those who want to receive letters have them forwarded on to the family. Very distraught families who cannot accept the death of their loved ones do not want to hear

Ruth Macklin

about the other family who the donation helped to save a life, or help someone see. I don?
know whether there were any letters of thanks to be forwarded on to me as I have move
and lost contact with the lady of the transplant team. I do wish the recipient has had a
better life than they had before the transplant and hope they are still in the land of the
living.

From all the stress from all the upheaval in my life my health began to suffer. I would
go to the doctor for help but most of the time it was guess work. Try this tablet or that
tablet. Some of the tablets made the first problem worse. I know the doctors tried with all
their tests and x-rays but I didn't improve with them. I had a few operations to have a clot
removed from my finger, a painful lump removed from my wrist, muscle samples taken
from my leg, during a pap smear test I was sent to a specialist for further investigation
and before long I was under the knife once again.

Two weeks after Jody's death I had to go to the dentist to have my lower gum sliced
open, the bone trimmed with a pair of cutters and filed level before the skin was sewn
shut. This was completed while I sat in the chair.

"Do you have someone to drive you home?" The dentist asked. I shook my head to let
him know I didn't have anyone to drive me.

"I'll be fine,"I mumbled. The dentist looked as though he thought I would not be able
to drive the car.

Ruth Macklin

"How far do you have to go?"

"Seven kilometres."

The dentist gave me a script to get medication to stop an infection along with his card on which was his phone number in the event the gum decided to bleed during the night. He watched to see if I would collapse to the floor when I stood up from the chair. With my spine straight to show I could do this I walked from the room on jelly legs. Made it to the chemist to get my script then drove myself home to bed. I stayed there until the time came to feed the animals. I didn't have to call him out during the night.

I carried on with my life under sufferance until the time to go to the hospital to have my hysterectomy. After the operation I began to think I need another change of direction in my life. There had to be a change to my way of living or I would not be here now to be explaining my life. I had decided to sell up and move to Bundaberg. To get away from all the hard work and finally have a rest to try to regain some semblance to my life. Once I had decided there was not turning back. Time to sit and contemplate helps you think there is more to life than work and pain. I had done my time and now I believed it should be my time to have a more quiet life.

As my father had retired from work because of ill health I felt it was too much to expect him to try to help me with the animals and other work. Not that my father seemed to have retired because there were always friends, or other people, arriving on his door step wanting him to fix things. He was not getting the rest he should have been having.

Ruth Macklin

So my parents decided to move to Bundaberg with me.

While we were in Bundaberg for a funeral my mother and I found a picture of a house we thought would be good for us to buy. Michelle and I drove to the address to see what the house looked like and the condition it was in. We knocked on the door and explained to the owner we were interested in looking at the house. He showed Michelle and I through the house. It seemed to be just what we were looking for. A place where we could all live but not be in each others pocket if we wanted time to ourselves.

"Would it be possible if I could bring my mother back to have a look through the house? My parents will have to approve if the house is acceptable to them as we are buying a house together. We only have today to look as we return home to Sarina in the morning."

"That will be fine."

Not long after leaving the house I arrived with my mother and a couple of aunts to have a look through the house. My mother agreed the house would be ideal. Close to the doctors and shops. Not out of town like most of the others we had been to see. With this house we would be able to share not have to drive from house to house if someone became sick, or went away. There would be someone at the house all the time.

"I will contact my agent when I get home to send through an offer to your agent. You should receive the offer in the next couple of days," I told the owner as we were leaving the house.

The only fly in the ointment was my parents had to put their house on the market to have it sold. Mine had all ready been put up for sale and there had been a few buyers looking at the house.

I had all ready started to pack my things in boxes ready for the shift when the house was sold. I don't know if it was all the lifting, or bending, but I began to get pains in my right side and become sick. So I had to fit in an appointment to the doctor, a scan and an appointment with a specialist who advised me I had to have another operation to have the floating stones removed from my gallbladder. Here I go again flashed through my mind.

"When can the operation be done?" I asked, hoping it would be done before I moved.

"You will go on the waiting list so I don't know when it will be. The hospital will contact you once the date and time has been fixed."

"The reason I ask is because I am in the middle of moving house."

"Let us know your new address and you will receive a letter." Another operation I thought as I walked out to the car. I won't have too many more parts left in my body if the doctors keep taking them out.

The animals I owned were all sold so they would not be a problem with the people who came to look at the property. Darkie the cow had gone a long time ago because she was too much trouble to keep in any paddock. She always found some where to either go through the fence, or under.

"If you keep this up you'll become sausages," I told the cow the last time I had to go looking for her to return to the paddock. Even though I had added another piece to the

Ruth Macklin

bottom of the gate to stop her escaping she did it again. I stood at the top of the rise to

watch Darkie to see how she would escape this time. She lay on the ground to slide under

the gate. "That's it! You've had your last warning. You are going to be sausages,"I

grumbled as I rounded her up to put her back in the paddock.

I really think she had a death wish. Come Sunday the day to take her up to the

slaughter yard to be made into sausages she knew where to go. I opened the gate while

my father had his car park on the road to stop her if she decided to take a right turn

instead of a left turn. She took the left turn and a right at the corner and along the road

then took a short cut up to the slaughter yard at a run. Darkie stood at the gate waiting for

us to open it to let her in. I just stood there shaking my head when she rushed through the

open gate. We thought we would have to heard the cow toward the yards but she seemed

to know where she had to go.

The horses, pigs and all the other animals were sold or given new homes. The work

load became less as the days passed except for the mowing and the pumping of the water.

Most of the packing had been done and rubbish was taken to the dump. I had parked the

trailer at the back door to throw things in before I changed my mind about throwing them

away. Other things I passed on to the children or went to the second hand dealer. So every

thing was ready to move when a buyer came to make an offer and wanted possession

within the week I was ready to move out. The boxes were taken into Sarina to place in my

parent? car shed.

Ruth Macklin

We were on a tight time frame to get the houses sold and the money through to Bundaberg to pay for our new home. One the twenty second of October the money was sent through just after lunch then we had to drive all the way to Bundaberg. My father and a friend went in his car with the caravan behind full with all my mother? dolls, flowers and ornaments. My mother and I followed behind in my car loaded with boxes. We arrived just before midnight where I had to go the the bank to get the money out which I had to give to the owner of the house for the pieces of furniture I had bought from him.

He was waiting when we arrived to hand over the keys and receive his money. He had moved his furniture out during the day but he did not clean the house. The next day the caravan was pushed into the carport and I stayed behind to do the cleaning with the help of aunt Emily. Dust from the curtains upstairs turned the water to mud before falling to pieces. So I had to arrange for others to be made. A house cleaner to come in and to have the fleas removed from the lounge room carpet. We spent hours working on the car shed on the side of the house to try to scrape the oil from the floor where his car had leaked oil. Twelve litres of degreaser, litres of water and a lot of scrubbing helped remove a large amount of the oil from the floor. No matter how much cleaning we have put into the shed floor the oil keeps seeping to the surface. The house was clean and ready when my parent? truck load of furniture arrived from Sarina to be put into the house.

The rubbish trees which were in the garden were attacked with the chain saw to be taken away to the rubbish tip. Uncle George and Aunt Emily helped me take the trees

Ruth Macklin

away while my parents returned for the rest of their belongings. At least when the trees

fell you could see the front of the house. Most of the trees need to be planted in wide

open spaces not in small garden beds. We worked hard to get the yard cleaned. Most of

my boxes stayed packed until I could find furniture which could be carried up the stairs.

The hand rail on the stairs had to be removed to force my double bed around the corner

and up the stairs. My father worked on the gardens and my mother and I with some help

from aunt Emily washed and packed the kitchen cupboards so we would be able to cook

our meals.

We kept working to get the house and yard the way we wanted it to look except I had

to find time to search for furniture to come up the stairs before I could unpack my boxes

of books, ornaments and other items. I felt as though I was on the move all the time with

not too much rest. Fall into bed each night exhausted but not to have a good night sleep.

Nearly every night I was woken by some one calling my name. "Ruth. Ruth." I would fly

out of bed think either one of my parents were sick and they were trying to wake me. I

would make my way to the top of the steps to listen for the voice, or look to see if there

were any lights on down stairs, but the lights were never on. Sometimes the voice would

be male, then female. I'd go back to sleep to be called once again. "I'm coming," I would

say as I made my way to the stairs once again. Each morning I would wake up more tired

than when I went to bed but I had to put one foot in front of the other to keep going. Once

again living on my nerves with not much sleep.

Ruth Macklin

On night not long after we had moved into the house we had trouble. My mother and I had left to go to bingo and my father was watching television when we had left. Because of his hearing problem he had the television sound turned up so he did not hear when someone jumped the back fence to take his stero from the back veranda. Later he went out to listen to records until we returned home but his stero had vanished.

"Thought you would be in bed by now," my mother said as we came in the door.

"Someone has pinched my stereo."

"You're joking! Who would take it? How did they get in?" My mother thinking this was a joke but I could see my father was very upset.

I open the kitchen door to go out on to the veranda to have a look. Where once the stereo had been on the cupboard there was now an empty space. The thief had unplugged the cord to take the stereo and speakers. The police were called to tell them what had happened but weren't very optimistic the stereo would be found. Next morning the police were back to say the stereo had been found. Our new neighbour had found the stereo in the nursing home yard behind our houses. It had been placed under a tree probably to be picked up later.

When my father went out the back to work in the garden he found where the person had been. He had climbed over the six foot back fence, stepped through the newly planted lettuce plants without stepping on any of the plants. So we went looking for some way to close in the veranda without shutting out the breeze but protect the furniture left on the

Ruth Macklin

veranda. The men were soon at the house to put up a wall and door. The wind could still come in, we could see out but no one could see in, or get on to the veranda.

We thought that would be the end of the trouble but not so. A few weeks later we woke to find a few panels of the back fence had been kicked away from the posts. Maybe the same person had returned to do more trouble but found the veranda closed so kicked in the fence. So there was another job we had to do. We had to buy new bolts to re-fix the panel to the post. Added pieces of wood to the side of the brick posts through which were threaded a few strands of barbed wire making the fence higher, and the barbed wire a warning not to attempt to climb over into our yard.

"Why did you put barbed wire on your fence?" asked one of the workers from the nursing home.

"To keep the burglars out. People have been climbing over the back fence."

"Thought you did it to keep the oldies out."

"No. Only the unwanted visitors out." Next my father decided he wanted the carport turned into a shed so he could use his tools, and a safe place to put all the equipment he had brought with him, which had been stored in the end cupboards on the veranda. The week the carport was to be dismantled and the closed-in shed was to be put up, I had to leave to travel back to Mackay to have my gall operation. I went by train and stayed with Leanne for a couple of days after the operation before I returned home to find the shed in place.

After I arrived at the ward in the hospital the theatre sister came to visit me. "Don't I

Ruth Macklin

know you? Your name sounds familiar."

"I have been to theatre a lot of times. The last time was a year ago. I came in for a hysterectomy last February."

"Ahh! Now I remember. See you in twelve months time." She laughed at the expression on my face.

"Ohh! No you won't. I've move to Bundaberg so I won't be back." After the surgery had been done I only had a couple of very small holes, which had no stitches but was covered by a small piece of tape. Next day the tape was removed and no one would have known I had just been in to have my gallbladder removed.

A few days before I had arrived in Mackay for the operation my grandson Damian had been born. Belinda and Leanne brought him to see my in the ward before he went home.

Ruth Macklin

Chapter Twenty-one

Our life seemed to go reasonably smooth for the next few years with my parents taking off for trips to visit relations, or just for a holiday. We travelled away to attend weddings. My parents and I went fishing at different places but didn't catch much, which we could eat. Then my father brought a boat to go out on the river. Everything went fine until I had to be the one to go out in the boat with him. Out into the deep, deep water of the river, which I was not happy about. Not that I became sick. Just that I hated the thought of having to try to save myself if the boat sank, or toppled over as the fishing boats charger up the river to get in their catch to sell. The huge waves, which rocked the boat as we were pounded by each wave.

"Hang on. We won't get swamped. The boat will ride the waves,my father would tell me as I hung on for grim death. I could see us being dumped in to the water with no where to go except to the bottom. Where ever the bottom was."

Going up the river was a lot better as we did not get rocked by the fishing boats. The water was flat most of the time. I didn't mind when we went fishing on the Baffle years ago because the creek was not too wide and we had to row the boat. The water did not rush in and out very fast with the ebb and flow of the tides. Most of my concern about going out on the river was what happened if my father had a sugar turn, or one of his mini

Ruth Macklin

strokes. How would I be able to get the boat back to the boat ramp to get help? I didn't

have a licence to drive the boat. I could not see me rowing the boat back to the ramp

especially if the tide was on its way in the opposite direction to where I had to go. I knew

how to row but I would not have had the strength in my hands to work the oars for too

long. Arthur, as in Arthritis, would have been complaining about the work he would have

been forced to do.

   After some time my father stopped wanting to go fishing, or many other places

because he could tell he was not able to do the things he used to be able to do. I tried to

take on some of the jobs he had done before but most of the time I had to force myself to

do the work by gritting my teeth so as not to feel the pain. My father would sit to watch I

did the work the way he would have done it himself even though I had been doing some

of the work for years.

   "You missed a strip over there," I would get told. He would be shading his eyes from

the sun so he could point to the place.

   When you're exhausted, tired and in pain you don't worry if you happen to miss one

piece of grass especially if you are trying to get the work done before the sun drops below

the horizon.

   My father still rose early each morning to work in the vegetable garden before the sun

became too hot when he would rest. Many a time he would come in side with blood

running down a leg, or arm, from where he had over balanced and fell when he had one of

Ruth Macklin

his mini turns.

Then just before his last turn my father was out in the garden trying to dig up his patch of potatoes but it became too much for him to do. I sent him in side to have his scrape cleaned and a plaster put on while I slowly worked my way through the small patch to did up all the plants to collect his potatoes. We knew the work had gotten too much for him but he was too stubborn to admit defeat. Defeat was not a word he had used over his life time. He all ways found a way to do what had to be done. Never let anything get the best of him.

Toward the end we had to get a wheel chair to get him from the room to the kitchen as the mini strokes were coming faster. One afternoon when my mother was not with in hearing range my father looked at me and said, "I'm not going to make it this time." I didn't know what to answer even if I could get the words past the blockage in my throat. The look in his eyes told me my father believed he would soon die.

A couple of days later my parents went for a sleep while I went up stairs to have a read and a rest. During the rest my father had taken a larger stroke which had affected his speech and facial muscles. My mother knew we had to get him to the hospital. We knew he would not want to go to the doctor, or the hospital, as we had tried over the past couple of days.

"Ruthie!" My mother called from the bottom of the steps. I knew something was wrong by the sound of her voice.

Ruth Macklin

I came racing down the steps to see what was so urgent even though she had not shouted loud. I knew something had happen. The one with the problem I knew had to be my father.

"Call for an ambulance. Make the call from your phone. Your father has had a stroke."

I knew this did not bode well for us. Could see there would be trouble once my father knew the ambulance had been called. He would fight even in his state to want to stay at home and not go to the hospital.

The ambulance arrived a short time later to check my father out. Their decision he should go to the hospital did not go down well. He fought with all his strength not to be taken from the bed room to the ambulance.

"We cannot force him to go if he doesn't want to," we were told. "The only way we can do that is with your permission. In which case we will have to call the police to help use get him to the ambulance." They had tried to convince my father to go but he swung his arms and kicked with his legs. The furtherest they could get him was the hallway but he would not budge from there.

The ambulance officer had to make a call to get a couple of police to come out to be able to strong arm him to get him through the house and out to the stretcher. Once on the stretcher and strapped in my father had to accept he was on his way to the hospital. He wanted to die at home. Maybe he had a feeling the doctors would try to prolong his life and have to live connected to machines. The thought of all the machines Jody had been connected to must have still been in his mind and did not want the same done to him.

My father may not have known it but he had caused a stir in the street when the police had to be called to have him taken out of the house. "He would not go to the hospital," I replied when asked. "My father has had another stroke."

We locked up the house and followed the ambulance to the hospital. My father had been admitted for observation. My mother and I went up to the ward with him. When he was put in to bed he wanted a drink of water but could not speak so he pointed to his mouth. Having sugar diabetes my father was all ways drinking water. The sign said "Nil by mouth" so I knew my father would not be allowed too much water.

"Don't think you will be able to have any. I'll go ask the nurse." I left the room to ask.

"You can have some ice. The nurse will bring you some." As it was getting late my mother and I went home to find something to have for dinner and go to bed. Before that, we had to put everything back in its rightful place. Items we had to move out of the way so no one bumped their head on the ones hanging from the doorways.

The next morning we arrived at the hospital early to find my father had been moved from the ward to a room of his own close to the nurse's station for them to be able to keep a closer watch on him. He had become sicker during the night and had tried to get out of the bed. My father was still fighting to get away from the hospital. His subconscious mind telling him he was able to do it but his body was not able, the mind being stronger than his body.

Ruth Macklin

We sat with my father during the day watching him slowly slip away. When family and friends came to visit and began to talk about days long past, the fun and the hard work, my father would wriggle his toes to let us know he was still hearing what had been said. Until the last day of his life we stayed most of the day but had not long left the hospital to come home for our evening meal when the phone rang. No one had told us how much longer my father would live.

"I'm very sorry," said the nurse, "But you father passed away a few moments ago." He had waited until we had left the hospital.

"Thank you for ringing. I will begin to get things organised." When I put down the phone I burst into tears. The stress had been building for the past few days. I didn't have time for a full scale release of my loss as I had to pull myself together to make all the phone calls to relations to let them know what had happened.

"What's wrong?" my mother called from the kitchen.

"That was the hospital," I sniffed to hold back a flood of tears. I had to be the strong one once again. "Dad has gone. He died a few moments ago."

"We'll have to let everyone know," said my mother, as the tears began to flow.

I had just sat down to try to finish my meal when the phone rang once again. The call was from my cousin who had called in to the hospital to see my father but he was a few minutes too late. He was in his semi on his way back from Brisbane to Proserpine. He had detoured from his normal road to come through to see how my father was. Barry rang

Ruth Macklin

to tell us he had been into the hospital. He would ring ahead to let some of the family know what had happened.

A few days later family, and friends, arrived to say their last farewell to a brother, uncle, friend and mate. The house was full to over flowing with family who had travelled a long distance to arrive here. There were thirteen of us in the house. People slept where there were beds, and floor space available.

After every one went home I had all the leg work to do to notify government departments my father had passed away, getting his name removed from insurances and other things where the three of us were on together, and a hundred and one other things which I had done after Robert and Jody had died. Now I was faced with it all again. The stress had built so much as my body had begun to rebel. My legs had become so painful I could hardly walk. I had the feeling I would soon be forced to be in a wheel chair. My leg I had to lift with my hand to get it into the car.

I finally made some time to go to the doctor to find out what had caused my leg to go the way it had. The next I knew I had to make an appointment at the hospital to have physiotherapy to try to get my leg working.

"You'll have to go on a waiting list,"I was told, when I went to make an appointment.

"How long?" I asked, rubbing my leg to try to ease the pain from the long walk from the car to the hospital before finding my way to the physiotherapy department.

"Could be three, or four months. We'll give you a call when a space becomes vacant" .Fine, I thought, as I limped away to find my way back to the car.

For three weeks I had to grin and bear the pain before the phone call came. "We have some students here for a few weeks training which you can see. We would be able to fit you in by the end of the week."

"That will be fine. Any one to help relieve my pain." At the end of the week I went for my first appointment where I was accessed of my problem. My body was pushed, and pulled, until they finally decided to use the rack. Don't know what the machine was called but it reminded me of the days when people were put on a rack in the castle dungeon to prise information from that person. The physiotherapist strapped me to the bed, which moved. When a certain amount of pressure was applied I was stretched to re-a-line my spine. The treatment didn't hurt but it did help for a short time. I had to return a few time before I was able to walk without limping too much. I was given exercises to do at home.

As my stress level raised higher so did more problems with my health. Mother had begun to have more health problems and more and more work fell on my shoulders. Not that I am complaining. I didn't complain to anyone. May be I should have complained to release some of the tension and stress which I had suppressed deep down in side. Not sleeping properly was another factor of the problem. Not knowing what to expect but to be aware of what could happen.

Because my mother had a mole removed from her leg in the early 1960? and the gland taken out of the leg as well she became prone to blood poisoning. One moment she would

Ruth Macklin

be in good health then she would be sick. Many a night I would be woken to take her to the hospital. When I heard "Ruthie! I need to go to the hospital," I knew I had to move quick other wise I would not get my mother into the car before she lost the use of her legs, then I would have to call the ambulance.

First there would be the vomiting then the chills which hinted of what was to follow. The energy to the legs and then a red patch would appear to cover her thigh like the leg had been sunburnt. This redness would work its way all the way down to the toes before the illness went away, after a course of medication and a few days in hospital. Along with the illness the memory would go and my mother would wake in the hospital be to wonder how she had arrived at the hospital. So over time I learnt to sleep and listen for my mother to call but not get the proper rest my tired body needed.

One day I went to the doctor with an ear ache which would not go away in the hope he would give me something to take away the pain, thinking I had an ear infection. The first thing the doctor did when I explained my complaint was put the cuff around my arm to take my blood pressure.

"Do you know you have high blood pressure?"

"No,' I replied, thinking what had blood pressure had to do with me having an ear ache.

"Your pressure is 210 over 120," I was told. "Its a wonder you are still walking around. I'll give you some medication to try to lower the pressure."

Ruth Macklin

Stunned I walked out of the office carrying my scripts for all the medication to bring down my blood pressure in a hurry before I ended up having a stroke. For the next three weeks I lived in misery until the medication took affect. I worked during the day with a few spells in between but I could not sleep, even during the night. My mind would not let me sleep. I could not concentrate, or sit long enough, to read, crochet or watch television. At night when sleep would not come to me I would walk the floor, turn on the television for a distraction but in the early hours of the morning there was not much to hold my interest. I lived through the experience with little cat naps to keep me going. Once the medication worked and my blood pressure had dropped back down to a safe level I could concentrate and carry on with my work.

During the time of my high blood pressure I could not eat much food and I lived on fruit until I became over loaded with acid. I went to see my friend, Gordon, who is a naturopath and explained my problem to him. I was given a list of foods which contained acid, or had acid making products in them. My way of eating was changed and the stone fruits I loved to eat were on the not to eat list. I wondered how I would cope with the new list but I have managed very well over the past years. Do not even look to take a step back to the acid days which caused all the wind and acid to build.

Foods were not the only cause of the problem. Missing body parts had a hand to play in my health problems. You are not told, most of the time, what will happen when parts are removed from the body. Its not working right so the part has to come out, you get told.

Ruth Macklin

Each part of the body has a special roll to play to keep your system free from germs and clean the blood. When the gall is removed all the rubbish it took from the system goes to the stomach via a little tube, which will cause stomach acid to build. With the removal of other body parts you have another set of problems.

The removal of the uterus gives you another set of problems such as stress and menopause problems which you are not told about. "You don't need it any more," the doctor tells you. "You'll feel better once it is out." Why were we given these parts if they could be taken away with out causing other problems? May be they should have been made to regrow once the old model had been removed. A more improved model which would work better and last a lot longer if taken care of.

After awhile Gordon suggested I go to visit Bill, who does massage, to help me with the problem with my leg which had returned to slow me down once again. I made an appointment to go for my first massage not knowing what to expect as I had never had a massage in the past. Bill explained what he would do after he had asked why I had come for a massage. I lay on the table with a cover over me. When Bill was ready to start the moment his hands touched my back I nearly jumped off the bed. My muscles were so stressed the slightest touch had me jumping. Poor Bill was exhausted by the time he had finished because he had to try to release the stress from the muscles to help them work they way they were meant to do.

Ruth Macklin

Chapter Twenty-two

Bill worked hard every week until I began to get on my feet once again but it has taken me years to be rid of some of the stress in my muscles. I have had many visits for treatment, which makes Bill, Carol, and the rest of the girls feel like my extended family. After all this time, I can relax and Bill does not have to work so hard for the treatment to work. The crunch had to come for that to be able to work.

One day we had been out for a few hours at bingo and returned home. ? think I will go for a rest,said my mother, as she walked into the house to go to her bed room.

"I'll go have a read," I replied, as I made my way to the steps. I knew if I stayed down stairs to do some work my mother would not have her rest. She did not look a hundred percent. She looked tired and Aunty Phyllis had commented about the colour under her finger nails while we were out.

A couple of hours later my mother woke, sat up then made her way to the toilet but she didn't quite make it all the way. At the door to the toilet she collapsed to the floor of the laundry hitting her head on the wall as she went down. I heard "Ruthie!" moments before I heard the thump as my mother landed on the floor. I dropped my book to race down the stairs to find out what she had done not expecting what I found. My mother was

Ruth Macklin

on the floor laying on her left side, a leg tucked beneath her and blood trickling down the side of her face from the lump which had formed from the bump against the wall.

Shock hit first then the worry of how was I ever going to pick her up from the floor. I assessed the situation before I attempted to move her, or try to help. "You've done a good job this time," I told my mother, shaking my head wondering what I should do, and who I should call. I decided to see if I could make my mother comfortable before I called for help.

"Does your leg hurt? Nothing feel broken? Wriggle your toes." Didn't want to move the legs into a better position if the leg had fractured.

"Don't think so. Pull me up." I could see how uncomfortable my mother was but I had to be careful. I straightened the leg out in front of her with out any pain so I guessed there were no broken bones but a bit of skin knocked off. I took her right arm to help sit her up to lean back against the wall. To see what other damage I would find.

"What happened to make you fall? You didn't trip?" I asked as I applied a wet face cloth to her face.

"My legs buckled and down I went. Never had time to grab on to anything to stop me falling."

"This is an ambulance job. I can't get you up and you'll need to see a doctor."

I made my mother as comfortable as I could in the confined space before I went to ring

Ruth Macklin

for the ambulance. While I waited for the ambulance to arrive I rang aunty Phyllis to let her know what had happened and clear the way for the ambulance to be able to do their work and keep a close eye on my mother to see she would not pass out on me. Everyone seemed to arrive at once and the house became full of people and equipment. Once my mother had been assessed the time came to find out how we were going to lift her. Many ideas were suggested before we worked out what each one would do.

A sheet was placed around the back and under my mother's arms with a short length each side for the two ambulance offers to be able to pull. I found a low foot stool to be ready to push beneath my mother once she had been lifted to give everyone a rest. My mother could not help much because her legs were too weak. The ambulance chair came in next to be slid under on the next lift to replace the stool. Two pulled the sheet, two lifted and pushed at her shoulders while I had to be quick to remove the stool and shove the chair for them to let my mother sit in it.

There would be no way we could have taken her down the front steps. Lucky for everyone we have a ramp which goes out to the clothes line. My mother had to be wheeled out the door and down the ramp where the stretcher was bought around to the backyard to move my mother from the chair to the stretcher to be wheeled around the side of the house to be placed in the ambulance. We helped load all the equipment in the ambulance which had to be used. While the ambulance officers prepared to leave for the hospital I ran around locking doors, back the car out once the ambulance had moved out

Ruth Macklin

of the driveway and close the shed door before making a hasty trip to the hospital. I took the less travelled streets at a faster pace than I normally did so I beat the ambulance to the hospital. I had found a car park and was making my way to the emergency department as the ambulance drove in to deliver my mother to the ambulance bay.

I was allowed to go in and sit with my mother as the doctors and nursed assessed what had caused the fall. Test of all kinds were taken as I waited. Different treatment were given but my mother seemed to be fine until she began to slip away. She just seemed to be going off to sleep. A nurse came to check on my mother as I stood to pull the sheet over her legs which she had kicked off.

"How long has she been like this?" I could hear the panic in her voice as she double checked all the instruments.

"She stopped talking a few moments ago. I thought she had fallen to sleep."

People came rushing into the cubical and I was ushered out to go sit in the family room while my mother was disconnected from all places to be rushed through to the resuscitation cubical where the team set about resuscitating my mother. No one had come to tell me what had happened so I wandered out to find them working on my mother. Shocked faced shot in my direction as all hands stopped working for a few seconds before a nurse took me back to the room. My feet seemed to be planted to the floor. I was too shocked to utter a word as I assessed what was happening.

"Get her out of here," yelled one of the doctors, who were first to find his voice. He

Ruth Macklin

wanted me gone before I caused a scene, or passed out on the floor.

I had to hold it together. I could not let go of my emotions because I had to be the strong one who had to stand alone until the time had passed. I had to be there to be able to pass on what ever news, good or bad. The nurse took me into the room where I was asked to stay until someone came to talk to me.

"Would you like to call someone to come to be here with you?"asked the nurse.

"I should call my aunt to let her know what is happening." The nurse got me an outside line so I could make the call.

"I'm still at the hospital. The doctors are still trying to find out what happened," I told my aunt when she answered the phone.

"I thought you must still be there as there was no answer when I rang your number. How are things going?"

"Not too good. The doctors are working on her at the moment. Mum stopped breathing but they have got her back."

I waited for ages before a doctor came to talk to me. "We believe you mother has a problem called sleep apnoea. She breathes in oxygen to the lungs but she is not breathing out the same amount of carbon dioxide. The carbon dioxide is building up in her body which is slowly poisoning her. Not enough oxygen is getting through to the brain to keep the body functioning. We have had to connect your mother to a machine to breathe for her until this problem can be sorted out. Once we have her stable we will be sending her

Ruth Macklin

up to ICU."

"How long will she have to be on the machine?"

"Until we can get the blood gas level down and the amount of oxygen up to it normal level."

"Thanks for coming to explain this to me." I sat in the room waiting for them to have

my mother stable enough to be able to transfer her up to ICU. Wait there until she had

been settled then I dragged my tired, cold body from the hospital to the car to drive home.

Knowing my mother would not like what the doctor had done to keep her breathing.

Now, came the hard part of ringing all the family members to tell them what I could of

what had happened.

Not too many of the doctors knew about how the problem should be treated be it was

something which they had never came across. At the beginning the doctors had decided

my mother needed more care than they could give so it was decided my mother would be

flown to Brisbane. She would be taken to the Redcliff hospital because that was where

the specialist practised who dealt with respiratory problems.

Arrangements were made. Aunty Phyllis and I were to drive down the day my mother

was to go by air ambulance. The doctors and nurses had explained as best they could

what was to happen. I explained to my mother I would be driving down to be there when

she arrived. We went to visit my mother before we were to leave to tell her we were on

our way. I knew she would be in a panic. She had never been on an aeroplane in her life.

She would be scared. Also worried the hospital were sending her away without letting me know where she was being taken.

"We can't get your mother to settle. She's fighting the medication. We've just about to give her another lot of medication."

"She's frightened. Never been on an aeroplane before. Also she thinks you are trying to sneak her away without telling me."

"She picked a bad way to go on her first plane ride. Won't be able to admire the view."

So I explained all over again what was to happen. We were ready to leave for Brisbane once we walked out of the hospital. We would have a little head start on her but she had the quicker ride. Should arrive at the hospital not long after her. The machines began to settle to where they should be and the nurse was surprised.

"Looks as though she may not need the extra medication," said the nurse.

"She thought you were trying to pull a fast one on her." The nurse walked away shaking her head.

"We'll see you in Brisbane," we said then walked out to go on our long, nerve racking trip. To drive to a place where I was not used to driving and didn't know where I was going.

After hours of driving to get to Redcliff we finally found where the hospital was. We drove around the car park until we found a place to park the car. I was very pleased we had found the place without too much trouble. The next problem we faced was finding

Ruth Macklin

where my mother had been taken. Or if she had arrived for us to find her. Finding our

way to the front of the building was the easy part. We walked through the front door

wondering which way we should go. Looked around for some signs to tell us where we

should go. Luck was on our side. At a section just in side the front door was a Red Cross

information counter where they sold books, handmade clothes for babies and stuffed

animals.

"May I help you?" asked one of the cheerful ladies behind the counter.

We walked toward the counter where she stood. "We're lost." The lady smiled at us.

"My mother was flown down here from Bundaberg by air ambulance this morning. I

think she would have been taken to ICU."

The lady looked at the patient list to look for my mother's name. It was not on her list

so she made her way to an office to find out the information. When she returned with the

information she told us which direction we had to take to get to the floor of the hospital

we needed to find the ICU area.

"There is a buzzer out side of the door. You push that to let them know who you are

and who you wish to see. They will unlock the door for you to enter. You will be told to

wait in the waiting area if they are busy with the patient. The nurse will come to get you

when you can visit the patient."

"Thank you." We set off with a tired head full of information to wander through the
hospital.

We walked along corridors, up a lift and down some more corridors until we found

Ruth Macklin

what we hoped was the right door. There was a buzzer beneath an intercom system beside

the door. Phones at doors I knew how to handle. I felt like an idiot talking to an

instrument set in a wall. Anyone not knowing there was such a device there they would

think you had lost your marbles. I pushed the button then waited for someone to answer. I

expected someone to come to the door. A voice spoke to me from the box in the wall.

"Which patient do you wish to see?"

"My mother, Elsa, was sent down by air ambulance from Bundaberg this morning."

There was some discussion at the other end before a voice returned. 'I'll unlock the door

for you to come in but you will have to wait in the waiting room for awhile. The doctors

are with her getting her settled."

"Thank you." There came a clicking sound as the lock was released before we could

turn the handle to pass through the entrance. We walked a little way down the corridor

before we found where we had to wait. I nearly went to sleep watching the gold fish swim

in the tank, as we waited to be told when we would be allowed to go in to see my mother.

Finally a nurse came to find us to take us into the section where the patients were in their

beds. There was a nurse with each patient. Doctors roaming around checking on patient,

doing tests. When we entered the cubical where my mother was it was a shock to see all

the machinery placed around her bed to which she was connected. Small screens on

which the nurses could keep check of all the changes in the patient such as blood

pressure, pulse, oxygen level, rate at which the breathing machine (ventilator) had been

Ruth Macklin

set to do the breathing for my mother. Tube down her nose through which she had to be fed. A plug kind of thing had been placed in the main artery at the neck. A box kind of thing had been inserted into a main artery at her wrist so the nurses could take blood when needed to test the blood gasses. Another tube came out of her where the yuck could be cleaned from her lungs.

"We have not been able to get any response from her since she arrived. She should be responding,"the nurse told us. "Was she responding in Bundaberg?"

"She was given about three lots of medication to prepare her for the trip because she was fighting against the drug. She didn't want to go on the aeroplane. Thought they were sneaking her away without telling me."

"Ohh! That would explain why all her muscles are paralysed." We were lucky to get a room each in the old nurse's quarters, which were run by the Red Cross. There was a kitchen where we could cook a meal if we had time, or heated one in the microwave, make a hot drink. The rooms were nice and handy to the hospital and I didn't have to drive around the town. The car was put behind the security gate the day we arrived and that is where it stayed until the day I left to go home.

For three days my mother slept before the drug wore off enough for her to open her eyes. Three day she lost before waking up in a strange place. He life hanging in the balance until they could get the oxygen level to go up and the carbon dioxide to go down. Family came to visit and take my aunt and myself for short drives away from the hospital

Ruth Macklin

to have a proper meal as well as see something other than the inside of the hospital.

When my mother was coherent enough we were given a pen and paper for her to try to write messages to us as she could not talk with all the tubes down her throat. Then it came crunch day.

"The doctor would like a word with you," the nurse told me as we walked into the room.

The doctor turned up a short time later and my aunt and I were taken down to the waiting room where it was explained to us what he wanted to do.

"You know we can't keep you mother hooked up to the ventilator forever. She will get used to it being there and her lungs will become lazy. There are other problems associated with long term use. We have been gradually cutting back the amount of oxygen to get her to breathe on her own. Tomorrow we intend to remove the tubing. If she can not breathe on her own we will have to do a trachea to help her breathe as we don? want to have to put the ventilator back in. You know your mother could die once the ventilator is removed?"

I nodded to let him know I knew what he had been so tactfully trying to explain the situation. I couldn't see my mother wanting to be hooked to a machine for the rest of her life.

"Do you know what your mother's wishes would be? Do you have legal power to be able to make the decision about my removing the ventilator?"

Ruth Macklin

"No. This happened so sudden. No one has thought that far ahead. My mother has never mentioned what should be done if this sort of thing happened."

"Is there anyone else who may have legal rights?"

"Nope. Only me. My father has died and I'm the only child. May be you should talk to my mother to hear what she has to say." The doctor left us sitting there while he went away to have a talk to my mother. We never go to find out what, or how, the two of them communicated the decision, which was made. The doctor didn't tell us. If my mother remembered the conversation she never spoke of her decision. The look my mother cast toward the doctor when we were called into her bedside, I knew it was a sign, which told him to keep his mouth shut.

"Your mother has agreed to let me remove the ventilator in the morning," the doctor told us. "We'll have a team on stand-by in the case we have to do a trachea if she does not breathe on her own."

The next morning we were there early waiting in the event something went wrong as the ventilator was removed. The machine had to be turned off then wait to see if she would keep breathing before all the tubing was removed from her mouth. Then there was the wait for my mother to keep breathing, or stop. She was still given oxygen by a nose mask to help keep the oxygen flowing into her lungs.

The doctor walked into the room with a smile on his face and shaking his head. "She's a tough old bird. I think she'll make it. She is breathing on her own but she is still getting oxygen through a nose mask."

"Thanks for what you have done for my mother."I could have rushed forward and hugged him but I thought it would not be the done thing.

Aunty Phyllis went home by train on the Wednesday now the worst of the fight was over but I stayed until my mother was moved from the ICU into a normal ward. The move didn't go too well. Another doctor had to be called when my mother went into a decline.

"Can I see you out side?" We walked out of the room to the corridor was full with Christmas decorations. "Your mother has Phase Two Respiratory Failure. This means she does not have much more time. She is going to die. She should not be resuscitated. " A great Christmas present, I thought. "When she is well enough she will be returned to the hospital at Bundaberg. I can't give you a time span of how long your mother will have."

On Friday my mother had settled enough for me to leave for home so I could have the house ready for her return. There were things which had to be taken care of at home. I had the car packed early but I didn't leave until after lunch in the hope the rain would have passed by the time I was ready to take the car out on the road and make my way home.

I had to find the security guard to have him open the gate so I could drive the car out as I didn't have a pass to be able to open the gate. There was a misty rain as I drove away from the Redcliff hospital. The traffic was not too bad at that time and I did take one wrong turn at a round about by the road took me toward the way I wanted to go. It was a old

Ruth Macklin

back road which used to be the highway before the free-way had been made. When I

arrived at the town I knew which road to take to get on to the free-way to take me home.

The trip home on my own was long, wet, boring and I was exhausted by the time I

reached home as the sun was on its way to bed.

Ruth Macklin

Chapter Twenty-three

Over a week later my mother was flown back to Bundaberg hospital until she was well enough to move up to rehab before being released to go home. All that time, I worked like a slave to have the house cleaned, dusted and the bed made. In between work, I visited my mother in the hospital. I became exhausted, tired, and my body in pain from all the work, all the walking from where I had to park the car plus the air-conditioning. My body does not like long periods in air-conditioning. The pain in the legs drove me crazy. Made walking a lot harder. I began limping. I also had to watch I didn't turn quickly otherwise I would have ended up falling.

I did fit in time to go to the doctor to have the problem seen to and was referred to a Orthopaedic specialist, did finally get an appointment to see him and had to have x-rays taken. Some will back in two weeks. An appointment time will be sent out to you." I'm still waiting. I am still having the problem from time to time. Only for my going to have my massage treatment every two weeks with Bill, or one of the girls, I would probably be sitting in a wheelchair. But I try to block out the pain as much as I can by keeping my brain active. Rub my muscle with different creams and oils to help with the pain. Can? use too many pain tablets because there are chemicals in them I cannot take.

Ruth Macklin

Long Hard Road

After about three weeks the rehab team had my mother back walking with a walking frame but she could not walk too far. Her dependence on oxygen had been cut back to a few hours at a time at different times each day. I couldn't see how I would be able to cope with this new arrangement. In the end I had no say in the matter. The hospital had organised for a machine to be sent to the house for my mother to use. Someone was sent out to show me how to work the machine and I was told to go pick my mother up from the ward to take her home.

I could have sat down and bawled my eyes out. Here I had all this responsibility cast on my shoulders. A lay person with very little medical knowledge to be cast in the roll as nurse as well as do all the other work as well. There was extra work going out to find a stool for the shower and have rails put in the bathroom and toilet. A walker to help my mother walk. A chair to put over the toilet seat to make it higher and easier for her to get up without help.

For the first week I became exhausted and tired from all the broken sleep. My mother could get out of bed to make her way to the toilet but because of the low seat she didn't have the strength in the leg to stand. "Ruthie. I need a hand," my mother would call out. I would have to crawl from my bed to walk down fifteen steps to get to the toilet, grab her by both hands to pull her up, then trudge all the way back up stairs to bed. Half the time I felt as though I was doing it in my sleep. How I never fell down the steps was a miracle. My friends up high must have been watching over me.

Ruth Macklin

At the beginning my mother could do some of the cooking but in the end she could not stand too long to be able to do the work. She could sit to peel and chop the food which was a help. Some times that made more work for me when she decided she would like to make some pickles, or jam, with the excess fruit and vegetables we won as prizes at hoy. I had become the work horse with no time off for good behaviour. I wasn't getting a full night? sleep. I would just a tired when I climbed out of be as I was when I crawled into bed. Living on my nerves. Had to fight back the tears I could have cried by the bucket loads but knew I had to hold them back.

There were also quick trips during the day, or night, to get my mother to the hospital when she call out for me to rush her to the hospital. She would be in reasonable health one moment then she would get the cold shivers, begin vomiting, and I knew to run. Those were the first signs she was getting blood poisoning, or what ever the fancy other name the doctors have for it. The first to go is the use of the legs then the mind. In the end I had clothes ready to throw on as I climbed from the bed, rush down the steps and get my mother into the car before she could not walk. If I was not quick enough, or she left it to late, the ambulance would have to be called.

Then one Christmas holidays when Leanne, Shane, Mitchell Jack and Michelle were there she got sick. Thinking she may have been getting blood poisoning we put her into the car and I rushed her to the hospital. "Think it is a case of food poisoning," we were told. "There is usually a lot of that going around this time of the year." We were sent

Ruth Macklin

home. During the night my mother became sicker and weaker. I rang the ambulance

because there was no way we could take he safely down the steps to the car.

Blood tests were taken as well as x-rays and scans but no one could find what the

cause could be. The colour of the stuff she brought up gave me a hint of what I thought

the problem may be. "I think its gall stones," I told the doctors.

"No," I was told. "We've done all the tests but they don't show gall stones are the

problem."

My mother was admitted to the ward as she was slowly going down hill. The surgeon

became worried because he had no idea what to do. Because of the lung problem, the

doctors were worried about doing an operation in the event my mother died on the table. I

kept persisting it was gall stones. One hint was I had mine removed and a few of my

mother's sisters had to have their gall out. "This type of thing does not run in families,"

came the reply, when I expanded on the theory.

On New Years day my mother had been rushed down to have another scan done

because the doctors knew they were about to loose my mother. Luck would have it I

stayed home while every one else went out. "I'll will have a rest," I told them.

I had not been on the bed long before the phone rang. A few moments sleep would

have been good. "Hello," I said, thinking it would be someone looking for Leanne or
Michelle.

"This is one of the doctors who has been looking after you mother. We have done another scam which has picked up a blockage in her stomach. We are going to operate.

How long will it take you to get to the hospital?"

"Ten minutes. Less if I can by pass all the traffic."

"Come straight up to the ward. We'll be waiting." I rushed down the steps. Quickly

scribbled a note to say where I had taken off to and why. Grabbed my purse and car key

as I made my way to the door to the shed. In under Ten minutes I had arrived at the ward.

Lucky I had no traffic hold up and found a close park. Rushed through the hospital, up in

the lift and to the room where my mother was. I rushed into the room while the two

surgeons were explaining what they intended to do. Mum had just signed the paper for

them to operate.

"Are you the lady I just spoke to? Ruth?"

"Yes." He looked at his watch and shook his head.

"Took a short cut. No traffic to slow me down."

"We're about to rush your mother to surgery. We have found a blockage but not sure

where, or what it is. The blockage has to be removed. You can talk to her while we go get

everything ready to operate."

"I still say you will find it will be the gall causing the problem." The both of them

shook their head as if to say she doesn't know what she's talking about. The doctors

believed they would find a different problem.

                              Ruth Macklin

Everyone had arrived at the hospital to sit with me while we waited for the operation to be done. The younger of the two surgeons came striding toward us about an hour later with a bottle in his hand and a smile on his face.

"You were right," the doctor told me as he held the bottle out for me to take. "A gall stone was the problem. It had made a tunnel from the gallbladder to the small bowel where the stone became stuck. We didn't remove the gallbladder because it would be too long under anaesthetic for your mother. They will bring her down to ICU shortly."

"Thanks for coming to tell us," I told him. Surprised a doctor would confirm I had been right.

We all gawked at the size of the rock which the doctor had given to me in the specimen bottle. The ugly looking dark coloured stone which had been the cause of all the problems. It still is a talking piece today. If I hadn't persisted the doctors may not have found it in time. The operation was the last option to open my mother up to find the cause. The risk was very great for everyone.

My mother was kept in ICU for over a week before being returned to the ward then to home. Each time she came home from the hospital the longer she spent on the oxygen machine until she could not do without it. With each trip to the hospital I learnt more and more about what signs to look for for the blood poisoning so I was able to explain what the problem was. What all her medical problems were.

"How do you know what is wrong?" I would be asked. I would explain all the facts

Ruth Macklin

and show them the red mark on the thigh which was headed toward the toes. The redness

looked like someone had poured hot water on the leg, or had been too long in the sun. I

could tell them how I knew the oxygen level had dropped. I had all the medical jargon in

my head which some of it had been explained to my by specialists.

My mother was becoming worse by each day. I had more and more work to do once

she became incontinent. I was forever washing clothes, bedding, chair covers and the

floor. Most days I followed my mother with a mop where ever she went. I went out to buy

nappy like wear for my mother to use but sometimes she left it too late to make her way

slowly to the toilet. This was not only stressful but I was slowly coming to the end of my

rope. To the point of a nervous breakdown. Or taking a long walk off a short pier. There

was not a part in my body which was not sore, or very painful. My brain was on the verge

of over load. I felt sorry for my old computer when I put too much on it and it became

overloaded. I may have cursed it at the time but without the computer to take my mind off

of my worries I may have gone under. I started going through some of my old stories to

re-write them. I printed out photographs of family members.

Then came the day which changed things for me. One morning we had just finished

breakfast when my mother got up to make her way to the toilet. She didn't look too steady

on her legs even though she had the walker to lean on. At an awkward place in the

kitchen her legs refused to walk any further. I quickly grabbed a chair to shove beneath

her before her knees buckled and there she stayed. No matter how much I tried she could

Ruth Macklin

not stand. There was no strength in her legs. On one side of her was the fridge and the other the stove.

The only way I could get through to the phone was through the lounge room where I had to move furniture to get there. I called the ambulance to come to take my mother to the hospital. That was the last time she came home. I could no longer take full responsibility for her care. The job had been 24/7 for over three years. She spent a couple of weeks on the ward and then the hospital rang late one Friday afternoon for me to come to the hospital to take my mother home. I arrived there to find her in a panic. She knew in herself she was not fit enough to be discharged. Couldn't do anything to help herself. Couldn't sit up in the bed without help. She was going blue around the lips and her fingers were also blue. The stress had lowered her oxygen level.

I paced back and forth in the ward not knowing what to do. I knew there was not way I would even get her out of the car when we arrived home. "You can't take your mother home in her condition," said a couple of the patients. "I would refuse to take her."

Another doctor was called in to okay it was fine for her to stay in hospital because the one who had been treating her had signed her out to go home. After a few my mother had settled once again and she was transferred to rehab for awhile. I tried to explain to everyone I was not in a fit state to look after my mother any longer. My own health had shot to pieces. All I wanted to do was cry. I could hardly walk and was wobbly on my feet.

Ruth Macklin

My mother was kept in hospital until she was assessed for nursing home care. She would be kept in rehab until a place became available for her once the assessment had been done to know which level of care she would need. The level was classed as high care. Then came all the paper work. I think I filled out about twelve trees of paperwork. Luck was on my side as the Social Worker helped me as much as she could as I had no idea what had to be done to have my mother put in a home. She was not very happy to be going there but she knew I was sick and needed to rest.

One day a couple of months later the hospital had found a place who would take her for a ten day in rest care to have a break from the hospital. On the day of the move to the home I went up to the hospital to pack all her clothes to be ready for the ambulance to arrive. While I sat there waiting a call came from the nursing home to say they had a vacancy if we want to have a permanent place. I agreed we would take the place.

While I waited for the ambulance to arrive I carried all my mother? belonging down to the car except for a change of nightwear in case there was a mistake and the nurses would have to change her clothes. The change of clothes had to be made just before the ambulance arrived. My mother was loaded on to the gurney to be wheeled down to the ambulance. I walked down with them so my mother would know I knew what was happening.

I beat the ambulance out to the nursing home and was carrying in all the stuff I had carried out to the car. The only park I could get was out near the road as all the parks

Ruth Macklin

inside were taken. Trying to carry a lot of things in the heat and not feeling well my legs became very painful. I had been at the hospital since early morning and now it was mid afternoon and I had not had a change to grab something to eat. Well I did walk past the canteen but when there are many foods you can not eat you by pass until you can have what you can eat, even if you are starving hungry. I finally made it home for lunch just before three in the afternoon.

Once again I had to explain all the signs to the nurses so they knew what to look for to give my mother the car she needed. She was put in a room on her own but they soon found it would not be convenient to the shower. They would have had to carry an oxygen bottle with or trail a long lead of tubing from the oxygen machine to the shower room, or toilet. So a couple of days later my mother was moved to a room where the shower and toilet were connected to the room.

A nursing home is a place young, and not so young, should visit to see what happens to them from smoking. They may think it is cool at the time but they do not stop to think of the health problems which such a habit will do to their bodies in the future. The damage it does to the kidneys, lungs, and other parts of the body. New parts are not readily available to replace what parts have been damaged by smoking. Maybe some one should think of how to redesign the body so a new part grows to replace the old so it can be removed with out the person having to die.

Once the lungs are damaged the body does not get enough oxygen to keep the organs

Ruth Macklin

working properly. The blood does not carry enough oxygen to the organs. Not breathing properly the system does not get rid of all the carbon dioxide from the body when you breathe out. This stays in the body and the system becomes positioned with carbon dioxide. The brain does not get its fair share of oxygen and it begins to die. The carbon dioxide kills the brain cells. If you do not die before too many cells are killed you end up with dementia, not knowing who you are, or where you are.

I have never attempted to use hard drugs but from what I have read, or seen in a movie, I would say what my mother has most of the time is a permanent high. Most of the time she is in a world of make believe. She could see people, and things, which no one else can see. Dead people come to visit her to keep her company. Talks about things which have happened to people only she knows. The snakes and spiders she sees in the room. A cat which comes into the room at night which wets on her bed. Sleeps under her blankets. Crabs she tells us are crawling around in the garden out side her room. People walking around with their heads chopped off. Most times the stories are so convincing you begin to believe her.

"Can't you see them? There over there. How much money did you father give you when he was here?"

"He didn't give me any," I replied, because my father had been dead for years.

"Of course he did. I seen him give it to you. You don't believe me,"she would finally say, when she could see we didn't believe her.

Ruth Macklin

"Where did he get the money from?" we would ask.

"There's plenty of money in heaven." Once my mother even had us feeding pretend mice biscuit crumbs under the bed. Another time a little bird she thought sat on the raining of the bed. A little girl sat on the ceiling fan in the room. Someone cooked cakes in the light socket above the bed. She could tell us all about the cakes. How the cakes looked and smelt.

Now she can not get out of bed because she doesn't have the strength. Once she used to sit out in the chair to crochet but she has lost all interest in something she loved to do. She can do imaginary crocheting when her oxygen levels get down too low. The last time my mother sat in the chair she had a fall. I had been to see her. The nurse had just wheeled her from the shower to put her in the chair. We talked for awhile then I left. I had been only gone about ten minutes when aunty Phyllis arrived to visit to find my mother had fallen. It was her fault.

"I had been sitting there a long time. They wouldn't put me back to bed," she complained, when she had her senses back the next day.

"No you hadn't," I told her. "I had only left ten minutes when you tried to put yourself back to bed."

"Well they wouldn't come to put me to bed," she complained.

"No. You thought you had been sitting there too long."

"My foot slipped on the blanket."

Ruth Macklin

I went on to explain I had come back to see her and sat with her for the rest of the afternoon after I had found out what had happened. A large black, egg like lump was on her forehead. A couple of cuts had plaster covering them. An ice pack sat over the egg to try to get the swelling down. The whole day was lost. My mother didn't remember I had sat there beside her bed all afternoon even though I had given her sips of water.

The only way we can keep our sanity and not break down and bawl our eyes out is to laugh at her stories. We take each day at a time because we never know what to expect each time we walk into the room. We try to agree with some of the stories. Some of the times we change the subject, if we can, so she does not get upset and stressed out. Being stressed makes the oxygen level go down because of the breathing pattern is forgotten and carbon dioxide begins to build. Breathing through the mouth is another problem when upset as the right amount of air does not get to the lungs. Nose breathing gets more oxygen to the lungs.

My mother has now been in the nursing home for over eighteen months where she has full on care. She is on heaps of medication for lots of different infections she gets. Continually gets a rash which does not go completely away before breaking out once again. The oxygen machine goes day and night. Some times the bottle of oxygen goes on as well as the machine when breathing is difficult. Ventolin is used to keep the lungs clear and help with breathing.

The level of oxygen can not be increased more that the machine is set at because the

Ruth Macklin

lungs will stop working. The lungs will think they are getting enough from else where so will shut down and my mother will die sooner, rather than having a little more time. But the end will come. I have been told a couple of visits ago by the doctor who attended to her. "You know your mother is going to die soon." I nodded to show I knew. "It is time to think about what you want to happen. What drugs she will be allowed to have to make things easy for her. I will send a letter to her GP to advise him what he needs to prepare for."

Doctors have been telling me this for over three years but my mother is still battling on even though she is in fairy land most of the time. It is like living with you head on the chopping block waiting for the axe to fall. I hold my breath each time the phone rings. Most of the time it is those annoying telly marketers trying to get you to do something you don? want to do. They must delve into private places to connect my mother to my phone. The phone has always been in my name only. Don't listen to what you tell them. Now I slam down the phone as soon as I realise who has rang. Telling my phone is for emergencies only don't even get through to them. These nuisance calls are not good for the nerves when you are waiting for the axe to hit. My life is not completely my own but I am trying to built a life where I have some out time while time passes.

Ruth Macklin

Chapter Twenty-four

Now it is my turn. Most every day I go to see my mother at the nursing home, unless I
am sick, or have an appointment which I can't break. I'm not allowed to go to see my
mother if I have some germ, which she may catch and cause her to get an infection on the
lings. I can't go too far away from Bundaberg because she panics and down goes the
oxygen level. Two times I was told to go to family funerals not far from Bundaberg but
my mother panicked both times. Many other times I should have gone further away to
sick, and to funerals but I could not go.

In between going to the nursing home I do my work and go to hoy for a break and be
with other people who have become close friends. I still go for my massage every two
weeks if Bill is not sick, or away. I won a prize to a free massage at with a lady but it was
different, changing the DNA. We had a good talk while I was there. Donna did help me
make a few changes in my life which I had not thought possible. She made a few
suggestion. I followed through on the suggestions.

"What things would you like to do? Probably a course to help you get started. Help
you get out there from all the stress. Do your own thing."

"I would like a good holiday. Would love to get back to my writing. And I need to learn more about my computer."

Donna made a list of how it would be possible to do some of these things. Suggested places where to go to do the courses. So I went home with my head spinning with all these ideas. I rang the U3A office to see what courses they had and how to join. Found out they were have a display of all the courses so I went along to see which ones I like. Which ones were the times I could attend. Who had places. I spoke to the people of the courses which most interested me. On my way out of the hall I signed up to become a U3A member. I was given the name of the lady I had to contact for the writing class. The computer class times did not suit so I had to look else where.

I did the first two beginner courses which helped but have not had time to go back to do some more. The first day I walked into the room to see the wonderful computers I was lost. My tired, old and overworked, Window 98 was very slow from being overloaded. The new computers were XP. So easy to operate and so quick. I fell in love with the computer. When I went home I dug through my draws for a piece of paper advertising computers. I rang to explain what I wanted. Not that I know much about computers. All I knew I wanted more memory space than I had on the old computer. So I asked for 712.

Within a few day I had my new built computer set up to practice on what I had been taught on the Monday before I had the next class. I am happy with my knew computer except for a few things which I have to learn how to operate, and find a good which I can use for what I want to do.

Ruth Macklin

For the past year I have been attending a writing class and have made new friends. I have learnt a lot from Diane and tried to do most of the work which had been set for us to do. It is not a boring class because Diane keeps find different ideas to keep us busy. We have had to do research to find the answers to some questions. We were given a lesson in writing jazz lyrics. We have attempted poetry which I had no interest in before starting the class. We do short stories. Each new project gives me new ideas for stories. If I didn't have other things to do I would probably be writing all the time, baring the pain when sitting at the computer for long lengths of time.

A few weeks before we broke for the Christmas break last year I woke in the early hours one morning with an idea which would not let me go back to sleep. I got out of bed to find some paper to write down the gist of the idea thinking it would make a good short story for children. The idea bugged me day and night for over a week not letting me get much sleep because the mind would not turn off. I decided to write down how I would like the story to start and finish. I began writing but the scene did not fit with the animals in the idea so I cast those few paragraphs aside to begin once again. Once I started this story had to be put on hold because the other one had taken over my life. I worked on it every spare time I could find.

The idea grew and grew. I had voices in my head changing the story all the time. Even when I was asleep the story line changed. The voices wanted to work when I wanted to sleep. Think they must have come from a different time zone. When typing out the story I

Ruth Macklin

would have the voices on one side telling what they wanted. Diane on the other side telling me the word they wanted me to use was not right. My fingers would stop as both sides argued while I though of a way around the problem. I would reword the sentence to make everyone happy until the next time.

In the beginning the story began with a family of four, mother, father, daughter and son going on a fishing holiday, as well as a kangaroo and a cockatoo at the place where they were to stay. Some where along the way all these other characters appeared in the story. When I finally got to the end of the story after about eight weeks the story consisted of over 61 thousand words. At the moment I am looking for a place to have it published. Now I am coming to the end, no, the beginning of a new way of life. I hope one day to have the money I need to complete my dreams.

I have been working hard as I possibly can to fit in all the different phases of my de-stressing program to help me get some of my health back, if not all. I have different types of musical sounds from Angel music, sounds of nature and Holosync sounds which I enjoy very much. Some times I lay down to listen and relax, then fall asleep. Sleep is what my body needs most to heal. When I am working on the computer I have the sounds playing through head phones which helps cut out much of the background noise which surrounds my home. At the moment the music helps shut out a fair amount of the noise from the build sight behind the house. The vibration from the heavy machinery drives me nuts at times. Especially the couple of weeks I spent a lot of time in bed because of a bug

Ruth Macklin

I had picked up.

I am also experimenting with different scents of aromatherapy oils to help clear chakra points to help the flow of the body, to take away the bad karma. Have spaced my work, rest, reading, visiting and writing so as not to get stressed. I find I seem to get more work done that way then trying to rush around from job to job which I found most were not being completed. Now I do a job then have a rest break. Either lay or sit to read, or work on my writing, while waiting for the washing to finish, floors to dry. Dusting is a pet hate because I end up sneezing a lot, or get Hay fever.

Menopause is another problem. I have been suffering with it for years but didn't know what I was suffering from until recently. One day I found an interesting children? move to watch, well listen to as I worked on a piece of knitting to get it finished before the Summer arrived. Every add break there was this add about menopause and some of the symptoms. They all sounded like what had been worrying me. I had been on HRT but when I realised the tablet was made from pregnant horse pee the tablets went in the bin. This new medication was said to be made from a natural plant. I love natural. Unnatural you never know which chemicals are slipped in to the tablet.

I wrote down the details. Later that night I did some research on the Menopause Institute of Australia on my computer. I sent off a request for more information leaving all my home details. I soon received a phone call to find out why I thought I had a menopause problem. My answer to most of the questions were yes. I was given a time for

Ruth Macklin

the doctor to ring to discuss my problem and how it could be treated. I agreed to try the treatment. Money was sent to pay for the medication one day and I had my medication a few days later. Each person has the medication made to suit their needs. It can be adjusted if need be. The hormonal treatment is working good for me. I have had the best sleep for years. My life has changed in the three months I have been on the program.

My eating habits have changed. My stress is slowly leaving and so is some of my weight. I all ways told the doctor it was not caused through the food which I ate. My problem was the stress. Now I'm de-stressing some of the weight is slowly falling away. May be in the future I will be half the size I am at the moment. I am very thankful for the support I have received from the Menopause Institute. Very pleased I was meant to watch the movie. Someone was pushing me in the right direction. Most times it pays to listen to unspoken words of advice.

One day I may be able to go for a very relaxing holiday. I could do with a holiday where I could do my own thing. Find a paradise where I can roam to look at the sights, rest when I wanted and look for more ideas to keep my mind working on stories. A place where I didn't have to worry about being at certain times.

In paradise I may find my Prince Charming who will treat me as his Princess for awhile before I have to return to my home. To return home to find out my next story has been accepted to be published, or going to be made into a movie. I feel lost when I have reached the end. I live the story in my mind as I work. It is like the house being empty as

Ruth Macklin

each member of your family leaves home to begin to have a life of their own.

Here's hoping in the future my dreams will come to pass. I will have the money to build and live my dream. To be there to help others who may find themselves in the places where I have been. To find more interesting ways of helping me keep the stress from my life in a natural way. That one day I'll truly be living in my dream castle. Living in my Castle of Angels.

Ruth Macklin

Chapter Twenty-five

My mother is no longer suffering. Living a life she was never meant to have. She had worked hard all her life, along side my father, to end up bed ridden for the final days of her life. Mum passed over on 1ˢᵗ October, 2009. Went to be with my father, and grandchildren, who went before her. She went out peacefully in the early hours of the morning.

The hard part, even though I knew I would have to make the tough decision, I had to give the doctors permission to stop her medication. There had been a 'No Resuscitation' note put on her medical record. I knew the time had come to let her go on her journey to a more peaceful life.

A couple of nights before she took her final breath, in my sleep, I told Jody it was time to come to take mum home to be with her and dad. I said the time had come for me to let her go. The next morning, when I went to the hospital I could see a different change on my mother's face. She was at peace waiting for her final journey to another life, to begin. On the day of her funeral, I walked beside the coffin when she was being carried out, to hand her spirit over into the hands of her loved one who had taken the journey before her. She will forever be missed by all who are left until it is time for our journey.

Ruth Macklin

My Mother's Farewell.

Clouds of peace rose from
the casket on the alter.
We stood as one
Jack and I walked forward
to place rose petals with love.
A mother, great-grandmother
had departed leaving this earth,
to travel to a land without pain.
Took our place of humour
beside the casket on this
her final journey.
Jody helped escort us
to the waiting hearse.
She gladly walked
her grandmother to the land
of peace and tranquillity,
where my mother now stands
beside my father for eternity.

Ruth Macklin

www.ingramcontent.com/pod-product-compliance
Lightning Source LLC
Chambersburg PA
CBHW060237290526
45789CB00001B/92